Computers for Nurses

AF526554

Computers for Nurses

Second Edition

Editors

Niranjan Shendurnikar MD FIAP
Consultant Pediatrician
Ankur Children Hospital
Vadodara, Gujarat, India

Naveen Thacker MD FIAP
Consultant Pediatrician
Deep Children Hospital
and Research Center
Gandhidham, Gujarat, India

Executive Editors

Manoj Ambwani MD
Consultant Pediatrician
Ideal Clinic & Nursing Home
Vadodara, Gujarat, India

Bakulesh M Chauhan MD PGDAP
Consultant Pediatrician
Manav Hospital
Vadodara, Gujarat, India

Foreword
Anita Deodhar

JAYPEE *The Health Sciences Publisher*
New Delhi | London | Panama

JAYPEE **Jaypee Brothers Medical Publishers (P) Ltd**

Headquarters

Jaypee Brothers Medical Publishers (P) Ltd.
4838/24, Ansari Road, Daryaganj
New Delhi 110 002, India
Phone: +91-11-43574357
Fax: +91-11-43574314
Email: jaypee@jaypeebrothers.com

Overseas Offices

J.P. Medical Ltd.
83, Victoria Street, London
SW1H 0HW (UK)
Phone: +44-20 3170 8910
Fax: +44-(0)20 3008 6180
Email: info@jpmedpub.com

Jaypee-Highlights Medical Publishers Inc.
City of Knowledge, Bld. 235, 2nd Floor, Clayton
Panama City, Panama
Phone: +1 507-301-0496
Fax: +1 507-301-0499
Email: cservice@jphmedical.com

Jaypee Brothers Medical Publishers (P) Ltd.
Bhotahity, Kathmandu, Nepal
Phone: +977-9741283608
Email: kathmandu@jaypeebrothers.com

Jaypee Brothers Medical Publishers (P) Ltd.
17/1-B, Babar Road, Block-B, Shaymali
Mohammadpur, Dhaka-1207
Bangladesh
Mobile: +08801912003485
Email: jaypeedhaka@gmail.com

Website: www.jaypeebrothers.com
Website: www.jaypeedigital.com

© 2017, Jaypee Brothers Medical Publishers

The views and opinions expressed in this book are solely those of the original contributor(s)/author(s) and do not necessarily represent those of editor(s) of the book.

All rights reserved. No part of this publication may be reproduced, stored or transmitted in any form or by any means, electronic, mechanical, photocopying, recording or otherwise, without the prior permission in writing of the publishers.

All brand names and product names used in this book are trade names, service marks, trademarks or registered trademarks of their respective owners. The publisher is not associated with any product or vendor mentioned in this book.

Medical knowledge and practice change constantly. This book is designed to provide accurate, authoritative information about the subject matter in question. However, readers are advised to check the most current information available on procedures included and check information from the manufacturer of each product to be administered, to verify the recommended dose, formula, method and duration of administration, adverse effects and contraindications. It is the responsibility of the practitioner to take all appropriate safety precautions. Neither the publisher nor the author(s)/editor(s) assume any liability for any injury and/or damage to persons or property arising from or related to use of material in this book.

This book is sold on the understanding that the publisher is not engaged in providing professional medical services. If such advice or services are required, the services of a competent medical professional should be sought.

Every effort has been made where necessary to contact holders of copyright to obtain permission to reproduce copyright material. If any have been inadvertently overlooked, the publisher will be pleased to make the necessary arrangements at the first opportunity.

Inquiries for bulk sales may be solicited at: jaypee@jaypeebrothers.com

Computers for Nurses

First Edition: **2006**

Reprint: **2010**

Second Edition: **2017**, **Reprint: 2025**

ISBN 978-93-86150-85-1

Printed in India

Contributors

Bakulesh M Chauhan MD PGDAP
Consultant Pediatrician
Manav Hospital
Vadodara, Gujarat, India
☛ *Computer Ergonomics*

Bhavesh Shah MD
Consultant Pediatrician
Riddhi Children Hospital
Vadodara, Gujarat, India
☛ *Maintenance and Taking Care of Computers*

Jagdish Chinnappa MD
Consultant Pediatrician
Manipal Hospital
Bengaluru, Karnataka, India
☛ *Hospital Information Systems*

Jeeson Unni MD DCH FIAP
Consultant Pediatrician
Dr Kunhalu's Nursing Home
Ernakulam, Kerala, India
☛ *Social Networking*

Lincy John
Senior Project Manager
Child Health Foundation
Gandhidham, Gujarat, India
☛ *Concepts of Computers*
☛ *Application of Computers in Nursing*

Maansi Ramnani
Assistant Project Manager
Child Health Foundation
Gandhidham, Gujarat, India
☛ *Multimedia*

Manoj Ambwani MD
Consultant Pediatrician
Ideal Clinic & Nursing Home
Vadodara, Gujarat, India
☛ *Selecting a Computer*

Mukesh Kumar Singh MD FNB
Pediatric Cardiologist
Kailash Hospital
Vadodara, Gujarat, India
☛ *Patient Education and Information Technology*

Naveen Thacker MD FIAP
Consultant Pediatrician
Deep Children Hospital and Research Center
Gandhidham, Gujarat, India
☛ *Concepts of Computers*
☛ *Telemedicine*
☛ *Application of Computers in Nursing*

Neelkamal Kapoor MD
Professor of Pathology
AIIMS
Bhopal, Madhya Pradesh, India
☛ *PowerPoint Presentation*

Nikita Thakkar
Admin Executive
HBS India Program
Gandhidham, Gujarat, India
☛ *Microsoft Word, Excel and Access*

Niranjan Shendurnikar
MD FIAP
Consultant Pediatrician
Ankur Children Hospital
Vadodara, Gujarat, India
- *Internet Search for Medical Literature and Resources*
- *Patient Education and Information Technology*

Nishtha Kathuria Juneja
National Program Officer
HBS India Program
New Delhi, India
- *Statistical Packages: Types and their Features*

Paresh Thakkar MD DNB
Associate Professor of Pediatrics
Vadodara Medical College
Gujarat, India
- *Internet Search for Medical Literature and Resources*

Pradeep Kapoor MD
Consultant Pediatrician
Computerized Child Clinic
Bhopal, Madhya Pradesh, India
- *PowerPoint Presentation*

Pritesh Nagar MD
Consultant Pediatric Intensivist
Aditya Hospital
Hyderabad, Telangana, India
- *Smartphones and their Applications*

Rajinder Gulati MD FIAP
I/C Medical Officer
ESIC Hospital
Ludhiana, Punjab, India
- *Backing up the Data*

Sachidanand Kamath
MD DCH FIAP PGDAP
Consultant Pediatrician
Welfare Hospital
Ernakulam, Kerala, India
- *Social Networking*

Sandeep Thacker MBBS
Medical Officer
Deep Children Hospital
Gandhidham, Gujarat, India
- *Telemedicine*

Sanjeev Goel MD
Consultant Pediatrician
Saakshi Children Hospital
Vadodara, Gujarat, India
- *Understanding Mobile Operating Systems*

Sumeet Juneja
State Technical Officer
Rotavirus Vaccine Introduction
JSI, Panchkula, Haryana, India
- *Statistical Packages: Types and their Features*

Upant Rao Dongre
Assistant National Program Officer
HBS India Program
Gandhidham, Gujarat, India
- *Microsoft Word, Excel and Access*
- *Multimedia*

Yatin Mehta DCH DCAH
Consultant Pediatrician
Sameep Children Hospital
Vadodara, Gujarat, India
- *Computer Security and Virus Protection*

Foreword

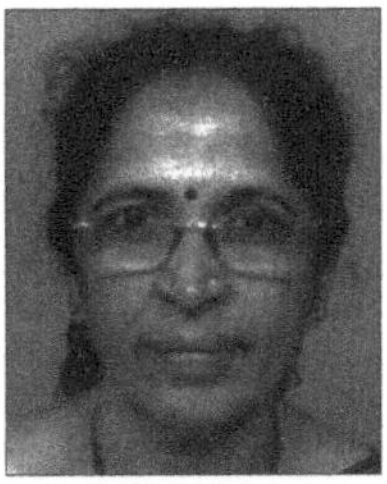

It is indeed a great pleasure to write a foreword for a different type of book, which is not directly connected with nursing and patient care. The world is now moving ahead with computers and it is a need of the hour for people in every field of life such as education, business or community living, to be well-versed with computers. The present generation is computer savvy because of the interest, good grasping power and practice, even though, many times, they may be ignoring the basic scientific part of the computers and computerization.

The editors of this book, Dr Niranjan Shendurnikar and Dr Naveen Thacker, and the team of contributors are experts in their individual fields. The book has covered all topics in computer management, right from selecting a proper computer, its security and protection from virus, maintenance and data backup to computer ergonomics. It rightly includes the important topic on how to prepare PowerPoint presentation, which would be of great help to student nurses during their educational period and further in their professional career. It also highlights easy ways of searching for the required information/ literature.

The book includes a separate chapter on smartphones and their role in forming the social network; how to make use of this tool for patient's education and information has been adequately described. An important and useful chapter detailing about 'telemedicine', which is comparatively a recently developed technology, has also been included in this book. Many hospitals and institutions may not have this facility, and as such, many nurses may not have any knowledge about it. The said chapter shall certainly help nursing professionals to know and learn about telemedicine, which would be a major requirement in the coming years.

I am sure this book shall be of great help to all and enlighten the qualified nurse practitioners and student nurses. The book shall help nursing professionals in cultivating proper rapport between the health workers leading to further improvement in patient care system.

Anita Deodhar MScN
President, Trained Nurses Association of India (TNAI)
New Delhi, India

Preface to the Second Edition

Since the advent of computers and information technology over the past few decades, these tools have become an essential and an inseparable part of healthcare systems. It is difficult to imagine the provision of healthcare without the use of these ever evolving gadgets. Computers have proven to be offering multiple benefits to the healthcare professionals—be in a rapid processing of the information or an improved access to the burgeoning medical literature, or an endless capacity for the storage of the information. Besides, the vast network of Internet and the expanding functional applications of the smart phones have brought the world on our desktops and within our hands. With such an ongoing and rapid pace of developments and increasing penetration of the technology, it becomes mandatory to continually learn and adapt to the computing world.

In spite of the need, there remains a limited availability of the resources on this subject for healthcare professionals and still less for the students and the staff of the nursing profession. The objective behind bringing out this book is to provide its readers an easy-to-understand, follow and practice approach about the unlimited usage of computers and information technology. Besides, the tools and technology need to be understood in their best perspectives if the user has to make its best uses and derive the ultimate benefit for the best of patient care in health systems. We do realize that a substantial number of the readers would be computer savvy, but for often overlooked basics, essential know-how, newer features and the ongoing developments, which form an integral part of the text. These features hopefully should make the book an important tool in the learning kits of the healthcare professionals.

We are extremely fortunate to tap the cream of talents of versatile experts who by the virtue of their hard work, passion and dedication in the field of information technology, have gratefully contributed to make the book what it is expected to be. Their expertise in the field of computer applications should prove to be handy and practically useful for the readers of the book. We are also sincerely grateful to Jaypee Brothers Medical Publishers and their dedicated publishing team for having belief in us and supporting our endeavor all throughout. We earnestly believe that with the continued expansion of information-rich healthcare and the society, the only way forward is to embrace this technology completely and keep in pace with learning its newer and ongoing developments.

Niranjan Shendurnikar
Naveen Thacker
Manoj Ambwani
Bakulesh M Chauhan

Preface to the First Edition

Health sector is one of the largest consumer-oriented fields, which can derive substantial benefits from the computerization. Last few years have been continually witnessing an increasing number of health professionals and setups, using electronic and information technology to improvise the delivery of healthcare at different levels such as primary care, ambulatory care and tertiary level care. Expectedly this advancement has revolutionized utilization of manpower, economic resources and brought about an effective and efficient time management.

Computers and information technology by their rapid processing of information, endless capacity for storage of information and an improved access to literature have led it to become an essential tool in day-to-day medical practice. The book has been simply written with an objective to provide an easy step-by-step understanding in making the readers aware about the expanded spectrum of computer usage in healthcare systems. The book should act as a good starting point towards getting to know some of the issues such as telemedicine and digital imaging, which though not widely available as yet, are likely to influence the patient care in near future. Especially for beginners, the book takes a simple approach towards learning and practicing important concepts related to searching information on internet, educating patients on health and preparing an effective audiovisual presentation.

Naveen Thacker
Niranjan Shendurnikar
Jeeson C Unni
Jagdish Chinnapa
Sachidanand Kamath

Contents

1

Concepts of Computers

Lincy John, Naveen Thacker

A computer is a programmable machine designed to perform arithmetic and logical operations automatically and sequentially on the input submitted by the user and gives the desired output after processing.

OBJECTIVES

After going through this lesson you would be able to:

- Familiarize yourself with characteristics of computers
- Identify the basic components of a computer
- Explain the importance of various units of a computer
- Differentiate between system software and application software
- Explain the importance of operating system
- Get acquainted with open source
- Appreciate the need of computer security.

CHARACTERISTICS

The characteristics of computers that have made them so powerful and universally useful are:

- Speed
- Accuracy
- Diligence
- Versatility
- Storage capacity.

COMPUTER ORGANIZATION

A computer system consists of mainly four basic units; namely input unit, storage unit, central processing unit and output unit (Fig. 1.1).

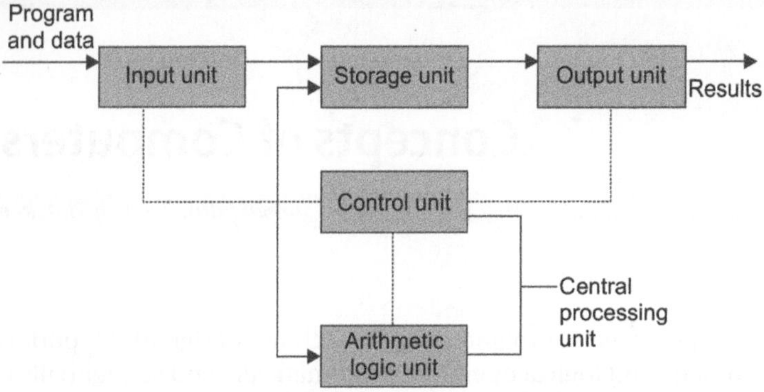

Fig. 1.1: Basic computer organization

FUNCTIONAL UNITS

a. **Input unit:** This unit is used for entering data and programs into the computer system by the user for processing. Different types of input devices are Keyboard, Mouse, Track ball, Touch pad, Touch screen, Light pen, Scanner, etc.
b. **Storage unit:** The storage unit is used for storing data and instructions before and after processing. Computer's memory is of two types; Primary and Secondary. Primary memory is further classified into RAM and ROM. Secondary storage devices are of two types; magnetic and optical. Magnetic devices include hard disks and optical storage devices are CDs, DVDs, Pen drive, Zip drive, etc.
c. **Output unit:** The output unit is used for storing the result as output produced by the computer after processing. The output is usually produced in one of the two ways—on the display device, or on paper (hard copy). Different types of output unit are Monitor, Printer, Plotter, FAX, Sound cards and speakers
d. **Processing:** The task of performing operations like arithmetic and logical operations is called processing. The central processing unit (CPU) takes data and instructions from the storage unit and makes all sorts of calculations based on the instructions given and the type of data provided. It is then sent back to the storage unit. CPU includes arithmetic logic unit (ALU) and control unit (CU).

COMPUTER SOFTWARE

Computer software is the set of programs that makes the hardware perform a set of tasks in particular order. Hardware and software are complimentary to each other. Both have to work together to produce meaningful results. Computer software is classified into two broad categories; system software and application software.

System software: System software consists of a group of programs that control the operations of a computer equipment including functions like managing memory, managing peripherals, loading, storing, and is an interface between the application programs and the computer. MS DOS (Microsoft's Disk Operating System), UNIX are examples of system software.

Application software: Software that can perform a specific task for the user, such as word processing, accounting, budgeting or payroll, fall under the category of application software. Word processors, spreadsheets, database management systems are all examples of general purpose application software.

Types of application software:

a. Word processing software
b. Database software
c. Spreadsheet software
d. Presentation software
e. Multimedia software

COMPUTER LANGUAGE

Computer language or programming language is a coded syntax used by computer programmers to communicate with a computer. Computer language establishes a flow of communication between software programs. The language enables a computer user to dictate what commands the computer must perform to process data. These languages can be classified into following categories:

a. Machine language
b. Assembly language
c. High-level language

Open Source Software

Open source refers to a program or software in which the source code (the form of the program when a programmer writes a program in a particular programming language) is available to the general public for use and/or modification from its original design free of charge. Open source code is typically created as a collaborative effort in which programmers improve upon the code and share the changes within the community.

OPERATING SYSTEM

An operating system is a software component of a computer system that is responsible for the management of various activities of the computer and the sharing of computer resources. It hosts several applications that run on a computer and handles the operations of computer hardware. Users and application programs access the services offered by the operating systems, by means of system calls and application programming interfaces.

COMPUTER SECURITY

Security has always been an overriding concern of human kind. For many organization, information plays a very important role in running business. Therefore, it becomes necessary to safeguard information from reaching the illegal hands. When data takes the shapes of digital form, a different security procedure is required. This branch of security is called computer security.

Information technology has many loopholes in it like stealing of vital information from one's computer or placing destructive programs in computer. The motive behind these activities is to slow down the economic growth of an organization. There are many such programs, e.g. Virus, worms, Trojan horse, etc.

Virus

Virus is a program which has been written to interfere with the normal functioning of the computer. It does this by clogging the memory of the system by making copies of itself or it may destroy critical information used by other computer programs. You can use an antivirus software to protect your computers from attack of viruses. Antivirus software falls into two categories: Scanners and Integrity checkers.

Precautions to be Taken against Viruses

- Install a memory-resident program in RAM that will detect and warn if a virus is present.
- Do not allow hardware engineers or sales persons to put a write enabled floppy into your computer unless they can guarantee that it is not infected.
- Backup copies of all programs and data files should be kept.
- Backup copies of programs should be held as read-only disks to prevent infection.
- At least two copies of the backup must be kept.
- Never boot your machine with a floppy from an unknown source.
- Always write-protect your disk when you use it in another machine.

FURTHER READING

1. Basic Concepts of Computers, download.nos.org/coa631/ch1.pdf
2. Wikipedia, https://en.wikipedia.org/wiki/Computer

2

Selecting a Computer

Manoj Ambwani

INTRODUCTION

In recent times, there is a choice of selection between different types of computers and these are of three categories:

1. Desktop computers.
2. Laptops.
3. Tablets.

All of these have their own advantages and limitations.

DESKTOP COMPUTER

A desktop computer is a personal computer that is stationed at one place and has separate tower, liquid crystal display (LCD) screen, keyboard and a mouse.

The major advantages of desktop computer are as follows:

1. Affordability, you can have a powerful desktop computer at half the rate of a laptop.
2. Upgrading and customizing is very easy.
3. Full-size keyboard and mouse are a blessing.
4. Graphic designers and a heavy gamer would always want a desktop computer.
5. No battery life problem.

Components of a Computer

The components of a computer you should know before you buy one (Fig. 2.1) are:

1. Monitor/Screen.
2. System unit, i.e. central processing unit (CPU).
3. Motherboard.
4. Random access memory (RAM).
5. Hard disk drive (HDD).

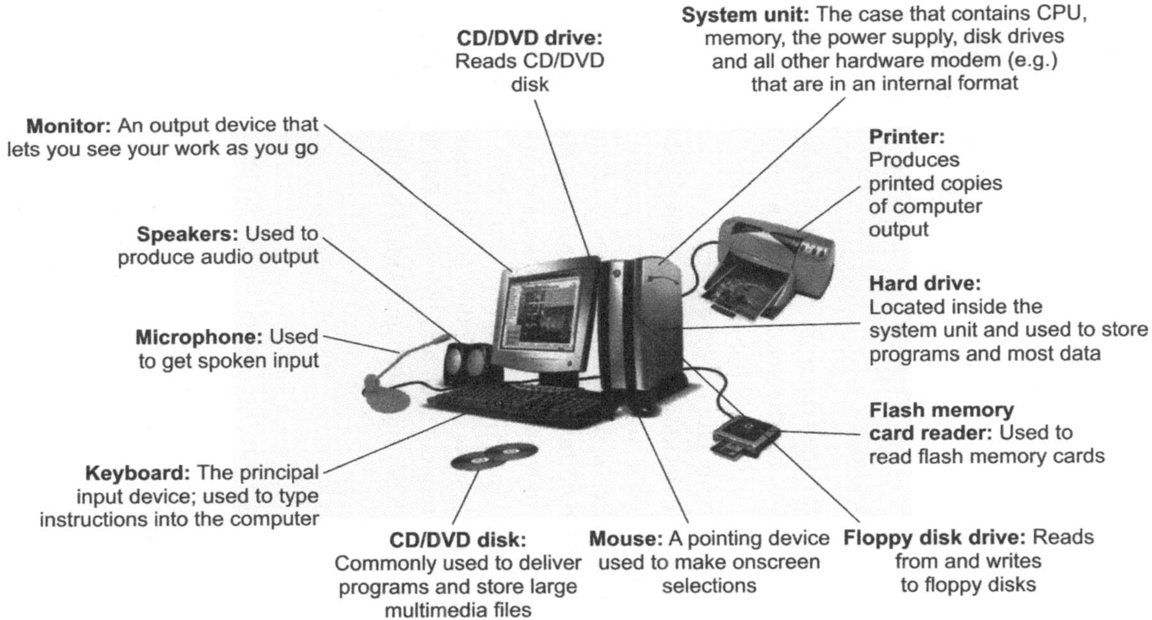

Fig. 2.1: Components of a computer (CD, compact disk; CPU, central processing unit; DVD, digital versatile disk; PC, personal computer)

6. Compact disk, read only memory (CD-ROM)/digital versatile disk (DVD) drive.
7. Keyboard/Mouse (with wires/wireless).
8. Multimedia speakers.
9. Microphone.
10. Web camera.
11. Modem.

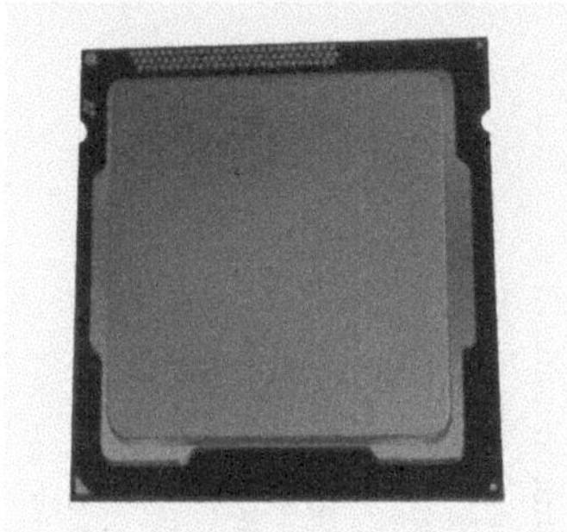

Fig. 2.2: Processor

Central Processing Unit

The processor is the brain of the computer. It is the hardware within a computer that carries out the instructions of a computer program by performing the basic arithmetical, logical and input/output operations of the system. When we are going to buy a computer, the first thing we need to decide is the CPU. We have a choice between buying an Intel CPU or an advanced micro device (AMD) CPU. If the price is not a restricting factor and you want to buy the best performance CPU, then Intel is the best. AMD has also been good as it is cheaper, only drawback is that it heats up more and is noisier.

The Intel Core i3, i5 and i7 are the latest from the Intel Corporation (Fig. 2.2). AMD processors are the other famous ones. The cost of an Intel core i3 is around ₹7,500 and i7 around ₹21,000. The AMD processors phenom II costing ₹6000 and AMD FX will cost ₹14,000.

Motherboard

The motherboard is the main circuit board of the microcomputer. The motherboard contains the connectors for attaching additional boards. It holds many of the crucial electronic components of the system, such as the CPU and memory, i.e. RAM, and provides connector for other peripherals such as video card, sound card, hard drive, network card, TV tuner card, etc. In short it is the 'mother' of all components attached.

The importance is that, the mother should have a matching slot for the CPU. Any motherboard will not work, if you are upgrading the CPU to the latest one, the motherboard also needs to be updated simultaneously. The CPU manufacturers are Intel, AMD and few others, while the motherboard manufacturers are Intel, Asus, Gigabyte, MSI, ASRock, etc. The cost of a motherboard ranges from ₹3,000 to ₹12,000 and beyond.

Random Access Memory

A random-access device allows stored data to be accessed directly in any random order. More the RAM, faster will be the multitasking of your computer. Nowadays 4 gigabyte (GB) RAM is the minimum requirement for smooth operation of Windows 8 operating system (OS).

There are few famous companies, i.e. Corsair, Transcend, Kingston, etc. With more RAM, the working becomes visibly faster and better. Corsair 4 GB RAM costs around ₹2,900 and 8 GB costs ₹6,480. Transcend 4 GB costs ₹2,500 and Kingston 4 GB costs ₹2,350. All these nowadays are, double data rate type three synchronous dynamic random access memory (DDR3 SDRAM).

In computing, DDR3 SDRAM, is a modern type of dynamic random access memory (DRAM) with a high bandwidth (double data rate) interface and has been in use since 2007.

Hard Disk Drive

A hard disk drive is a data storage device used for storing and retrieving digital information using rapidly rotating disks (platters) coated with magnetic material (Fig. 2.3). It retains its data, even when powered off. Data is read in a random-access manner, meaning individual blocks of data can be stored or retrieved in any order rather than sequentially.

The HDD consists of one or more rigid (hard) rapidly rotating disks (platters) with magnetic heads arranged on a moving actuator arm to read and write data to the surfaces. With an advancing technology, nowadays the hard drives of 1-terabyte (1TB) are available at competitive prices. Even those who want to have more space, they can go for external HDD, which costs only little more.

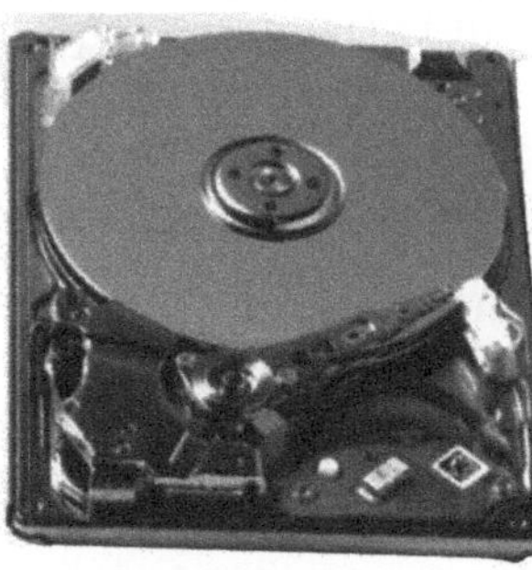

Fig. 2.3: Hard disk drive

Solid-state drive

The laptops have a solid-state drive (SSD). A SSD also known as a solid-state disk or electronic disk, though it contains no actual 'disk' of any kind, nor motors to 'drive' the disks is a data storage device, using integrated circuit assemblies as memory, to store data persistently.

The SSD technology uses electronic interfaces compatible with traditional block input/output (I/O) HDDs, thus permitting simple replacement in common applications. The drive have no moving mechanical components.

The basic need for more space is due to the larger files. A single movie in Blu-ray 1080p will occupy 15–20 GB.

CD-Rom or DVD Drivers

To install a program or to play movies and songs, we need the DVD drives. They cost around ₹1,000–₹1,500. A Blu-ray disk (BD) drive will cost more around ₹6,500. The storage on a CD is 650–700 megabyte (MB), while that on a single surface DVD is 4.7 GB (single side, single layer), 8.5–8.7 GB (single side, double layer) and 17 GB (double side, double layer).

Blu-ray disks

The name Blu-ray disk refers to the blue laser used to read the disk, which allows information to be stored at a greater density than is possible with the longer-wavelength red laser used for DVDs.

This is a digital optical disk data storage format designed to supersede the DVD format. The plastic disk is 120 mm in diameter and 1.2 mm thick, the same size as DVDs and CDs. Conventional BDs (pre-BD-XL) contain 25 GB per layer, with dual layer disks (50 GB) being the industry standard for feature-length video disks. Triple layer disks (100 GB) and quadruple layers (128 GB) are available for BD-XL rewriter drives (Fig. 2.4).

Cabinet with Power Supply

All the parts are housed in a good cabinet with proper power supply, preferably with uninterrupted power supply (UPS) backup, so that the data is not lost in case of sudden power failure.

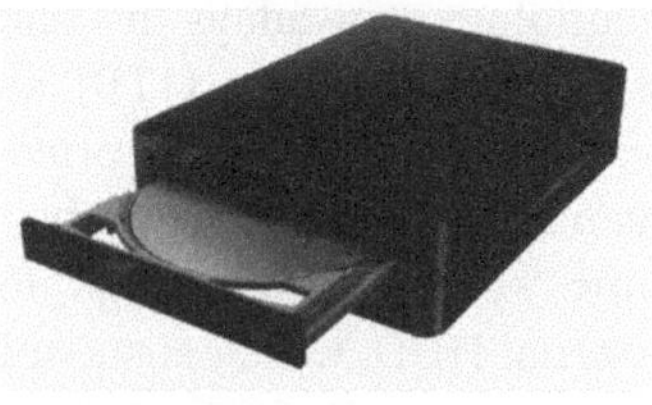

Fig. 2. 4: Blu-ray disk

Keyboard and Mouse

A cordless keyboard and mouse were usually expensive few years back. The benefits that are offered by these wireless devices are the convenience and the ease of portability. One can even use these peripherals, when the TV monitor is used as a personal computer (PC).

External Speakers

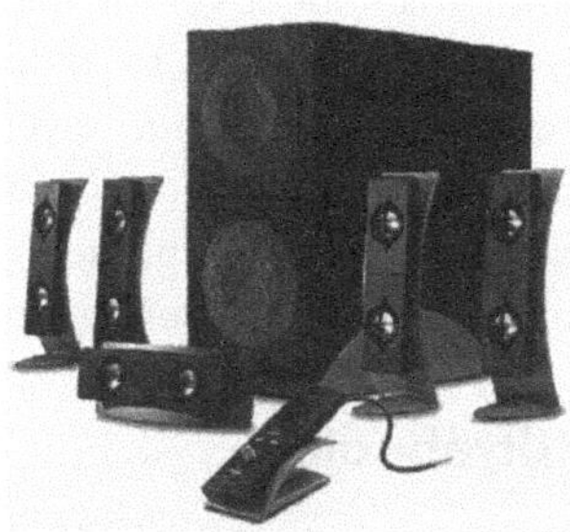

Fig. 2.5: Multimedia speakers

Depending on your choice, you can spend few hundred to several thousand for the speakers. Depending on the interest in music and creating a home theater atmosphere, one can spend any amount. The famous ones are from Creative, Altec Lansing, JBL, Bose, Logitech, etc. The ones, which occupy less space, are 2.1 format, where there is one subwoofer and two stereo speakers and they cost less than a 5.1 system. While a 5.1 will have one subwoofer and five speakers giving Dolby digital home theater surrounds sound effect. They are THX certified and have awesome sound quality (Fig. 2.5).

ALL-IN-ONE DESKTOP COMPUTER

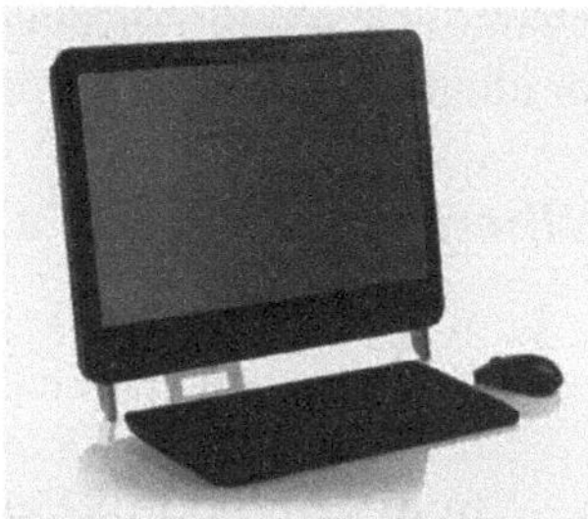

Fig. 2.6: All-in-one desktop computer

Nowadays one can get an all-in-one desktop computer. This has the CPU incorporated in the screen itself and all you can see is the LCD screen, and the cordless keyboard and mouse. It will cost more, but the space occupying will be less and there are no wires hanging around (Fig. 2.6).

LAPTOP

Standard laptops are mobile personal computers, which come in a wide range of forms and sizes (Fig. 2.7). They can sport displays between 10 and 20 inches in diagonal, they can weigh anywhere between light and heavy, and can bundle a multitude of hardware configurations and features.

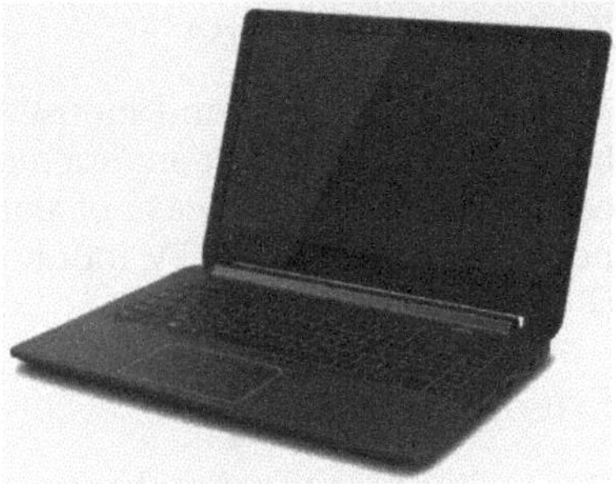

Fig. 2.7: Laptop

The 15.6 inch laptops are perhaps the most popular and cost effective, as they are powerful enough to deal just fine with all your everyday activities (browsing, chatting, listening to music, watching movies and playing some games) but also light and portable enough to be carried around when needed.

Ultrabooks

Utrabooks are a fairly fresh breed of portable computers. They are slim, light, sleek and fast that is why they will soon become more popular than 'regular' laptops. Ultrabooks need to be slim (18 mm thick or less for machines with displays under 14 inches and 23 mm for those with larger screens); need to bundle Intel's ultra-low voltage (ULV) hardware platforms and fast storage (SSDs or a mix of HDD and SSD storage); need to be able to run for at least 5 hours on a charge and support several Intel technologies, such as their antitheft or identity protection technology.

When will We Prefer a Laptop?

1. You are always on the go; that is why you want mobility.
2. Now you can get a laptop as powerful as a desktop computer, but expensive. Cost of a powerful ultrabook will be anywhere from ₹80,000 to ₹150,000. It is very lightweight, as there is SSD instead of HDD. SSD does not have an actual drive, so no moving parts and similar to a pen drive. But SSD is seven to eight times more expensive than a hard drive.
3. When we are always on the go, we want the laptop to be very light and hence, nowadays there is no DVD drive also.
4. The battery life, which is always problem in the laptop, as it will last only 3-4 hours. While in an ultrabook, the battery life is

double, i.e. 7-8 hours and would last for a longer use without recharging the battery frequently.

Limitations of a Laptop

1. Expensive to buy and equally expensive are the repairs.
2. Cannot be upgraded, except for RAM.
3. Heating problem.
4. Cramping of keys, as smaller the screen size, hardly any place for number keys.
5. Battery life is always a problem.
6. Screen size is a limiting factor.

TABLETS

An Android tablet is a communication and multimedia device that runs using an Android operating system. These tablets are the latest generation of portable computer technology with immense connectivity, capabilities and resolution. Steve Jobs was the one to bring the iPad in 2010. Tablets are small computers that consist of a single panel. Tablets do not have separate keyboards attached to their screens, as laptop computers do. Instead, tablet users operate the computer by pressing their fingers on a touch screen, which changes the views with commands. Microsoft released the first tablet computer in 2000. Android tablet computers began to appear in 2010 after the introduction of the iPads. Till date, 84 million iPad, have been sold in the last 3½ years. Overall, the sales of all types of tablets are much more than all types of PCs put together (Fig. 2.8).

The various Android tablets vary in their performance and features. However, they have common features through the Android operating system, such as a common management system for running and accessing application software (apps), which are software applications created for tablet computers and handheld devices. Android also manages activities such as engaging in multitasking work and navigating computer tools.

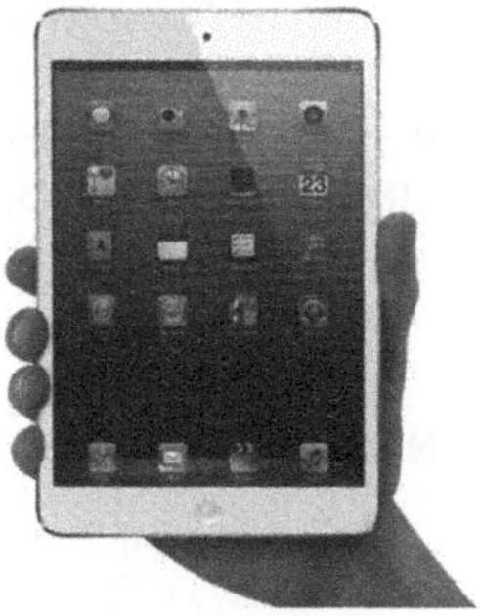

Fig. 2.8: Tablet

Advantages of a Tablet

1. Extremely portable, can be carried in your purse or small bag.
2. Not very expensive as compared to ultrabooks. Akash tablet promoted by the Government of India is available to students for ₹3,000. Otherwise also, one can buy a reasonably good tablet for ₹10,000.
3. Android platform or iOS platform have more than 1,000,000 applications to download and use for all the different tasks, games and entertainment.
4. Battery life is more than 10 hours and will easily last a day.
5. Can be used as a global positioning system (GPS) navigation device.
6. Connecting to internet wirelessly and surfing the net is a pleasure.

Limitations of a Tablet

1. Hardware prone to damage. If it falls from hand, it cannot be repaired most of the time.
2. No keyboard and mouse, so typing long letters or projects is not very comfortable.
3. Screen size is too small compared to desktop. So long working hours can cause strain on the eyes.
4. Do not have any optical drives, so one can never play a movie DVD or music CD. Connecting a universal serial bus (USB) drive also requires special cables.
5. Certain works cannot be done with a tablet; a full-fledged computer is needed for that.

CONCLUSION

Even as the technology continues to evolve and newer gadgets continue to help us making our professional work better, it is essential to understand some of the basic concepts of computing technology. Once when you decide the task that you need to perform, one can then make an appropriate selection of the right device in a cost-effective manner.

FURTHER READING

1. AC Mullick. Computer hardware. In: Thacker N (Ed). Computers for Doctors. New Delhi: Jaypee Brothers Medical Publishers (P) Ltd; 2003. pp. 10-27.

3

Computer Security and Virus Protection

Yatin Mehta

INTRODUCTION

In this era of information technology (IT), use of computers has become common in hospitals to store and retrieve patient data. The patient data is very precious and confidential. Thus it has to be stored properly and should be protected from prying eyes and also from damage by virus attack. Every computer has precious data in it and the one that is connected with other computer(s) or to the internet is vulnerable. It has to be protected from hacking and virus attack. The onus lies on the user of computer, to keep the data confidential and try to protect the computer from virus attack. It is worthwhile to know certain terminologies.

MALWARE

Malware is a term that is used for malicious software, which is designed to do damage or unwanted actions to a computer system. Examples of malware include the following:

- Viruses
- Worms
- Trojan horses
- Spyware
- Rogue security software.

Computer Virus

A computer virus is a small software program that spreads from one computer to another and interferes with computer operations. A computer virus might corrupt or delete data on a computer, use an email program to spread the virus to other computers or even delete everything on the hard disk.

Computer viruses are frequently spread by attachments in Email messages or by instant messages. Therefore, the users must never open an Email attachment unless he/she know, who sent the message or expecting the Email attachment. Viruses can be disguised as attachments of funny images, greeting cards or audio and video files. Computer viruses also spread through downloads on the internet. They can be hidden in pirated software or in other files or programs downloaded.

Worm

A worm is computer code that spreads without user interaction. Most worms begin as Email attachments that infect a computer, when they are opened. The worm scans the infected computer for files, such as address books or temporary webpages, which contain Email addresses. The worm uses the addresses to send infected Email messages and frequently mimics (or spoofs) the 'from' addresses in later Email messages, so that those infected messages seem to be from someone you know. Worms then spread automatically through Email messages, networks or operating system vulnerabilities, frequently overwhelming those systems before the cause is known. Worms are not always destructive to computers, but they usually cause computer and network performance, and stability problems.

Trojan Horse

A trojan horse is a malicious software program that hides inside other programs. It enters a computer hidden inside a legitimate program, such as a screensaver. Then it puts code into the operating system that enables a hacker to access the infected computer. Trojan horses do not usually spread by themselves, but are spread by viruses, worms or downloaded software.

Spyware

Spyware can install on your computer without your knowledge. These programs can change your computer's configuration or collect advertising data and personal information. Spyware can track internet search habits and can also redirect the web browser to a different website than you intend to go to.

Rogue Security Software

A rogue security software program tries to make think that your computer is infected by a virus and usually prompts you to download or buy a product that removes the virus. The names of these products frequently contain words such as antivirus, shield, security, protection or fixer. This makes them sound legitimate. They frequently run right after you download them or the next time that your computer starts. Rogue security software can prevent applications such as Internet Explorer from opening. Rogue security software might also display legitimate and important Windows files as infections. Typical error messages or pop-up messages might contain the phrases mentioned in Box 3.1.

Box 3.1: Typical error messages

Warning!
Your computer is infected!
This computer is infected by spyware and adware

TIPS FOR PROTECTING COMPUTER FROM HACKERS AND VIRUSES

Use Protection Software 'Antivirus Software' and Keep it Up-to-date

It is now mandatory to keep good antivirus software installed in the computer. All good antivirus software give almost daily updates. So check it that the antivirus program is getting daily updates and is fully updated. It is also advisable to do regular scheduled scan of the computer.

It is a good idea to install total internet security instead of only antivirus software. Because the former not only includes antivirus but also include antiphishing, antimalware, antispyware, firewall, etc.

Do Not Open Email from Unknown Sources

A simple rule of thumb is that if you do not know the person who is sending the Email, be very careful in opening the Email. If you receive a suspicious Email, the best thing is to delete the entire message, including any attachment. Even if you do know the person sending you the Email, you should exercise caution if the message is strange and unexpected, particularly if it contains unusual hyperlinks. Your friend may have accidentally sent you a virus. When in doubt, delete.

Use Hard to Guess Passwords

Passwords are the key to important data on the computer/internet. Passwords will only keep out of reach the outsiders if they are difficult to guess. Do not share the password and do not use the same password in more than one place.

Golden rules of password: A password should have a minimum of eight characters—use uppercase letters, lowercase letters and numbers, should have special character such as C5k$u8*, should not be a word found in dictionary, change passwords regularly at least every 90 days, do not give out your password to anyone; one can use password generator software for generating difficult password.

Protect the Computer from Internet Intruders by Using 'Firewalls'

Equip the computer with a firewall. Firewalls create a protective wall between the computer and the outside world. They come in two forms; software firewalls that run on personal computer and hardware firewalls that protect a number of computers at the same time. They work by filtering out unauthorized or potentially dangerous types of data from the internet, while still allowing other (good) data to reach the computer. Firewalls also ensure that unauthorized persons cannot gain access to computer, while anyone is connected to the internet. One can find firewall hardware and software at most computer stores nationwide. Do not let intruders in.

Use the Browser's Privacy Settings

Every browser has privacy settings that can be modified to make it more secure. This allows or disallows the website to use the private information. This is very important to prevent fraud and identity theft.

Turn on User Account Control

When changes are going to be made to the computer that require administrator level permission User Account Control (UAC) notifies and gives the opportunity to approve the change. UAC can help to keep viruses from making unwanted changes.

Let Not Any Other Person Access Your Computer (Log Off After Every Use)

The computer operating system may allow other computers on a network, including the internet, to access the hard drive of computer in order to 'share files.' This ability to share files can be used to infect computer with a virus or look at the files on the computer if do not pay close attention. So, unless one who really need this ability, make sure to turn off file sharing. Also when not working on your computer, log off. This will not allow any other co-workers access the computer without password.

Disconnect from the Internet When Not in Use

Remember that the digital highway is a two-way road. One can send and receive information on it. Disconnecting the computer from the internet when not in online, lessens the chance that someone will be able to access the computer. It is similar to closing and locking the main door of house, when you are not expecting anybody. Disconnect and be safe.

Backup Your Computer Data

If a virus destroys your files, at least you can replace them with your backup copy. You should store your backup copy in a separate location from your work files, one that is preferably not on your computer. So, all the important data should be backed up daily. Backup will save your system from any data loss in case of virus attack, malfunction, hard disk drive (HDD) crash, accidental deleting of data. One can take backup on thumb drive [available from 1 to 64 gigabyte (GB)] or on compact disk (CD), digital versatile disk (DVD) or external hard drive or on cloud.

Regularly Download Security Protection Update 'Patches'

No software is made perfect from the beginning. And so the importance of security patches. Regularly download and update such security patches for your operating system (OS) and for the browser (Internet Explorer, Mozilla Firefox, etc.) and for the office suite.

CONCLUSION

Keeping the computer safe, secure and virus free is just similar to protecting the home from thief and unwanted intruders. One should be prepared from advance. The antenna should always be on to sense the attack and to take proper action. By using common sense and caution, one will be rewarded.

FURTHER READING

1. Tips for protecting your computers from viruses. (2013). [online]. microsoft.com. Available from http://windows.microsoft.com/en-in/windows7/tips-for-protecting-your-computer-from-viruses [Accessed January 20, 2014].
2. Federation Bureau of Investigation (FBI). (2013). How to protect your computer. Available from http://www.fbi.gov/scams-safety/computer_protect
3. Western Carolina University. (2013). Ten tips for protecting your computer from hackers and viruses. Available from http://www.wcu.edu/about-wcu/campus-services/university-police/campus-safety-crime-information/crime-prevention-information/ten-tips-for-protecting-your-computer-from-hackers-and-viruses.asp

4

Maintenance and Taking Care of Computers

Bhavesh Shah

INTRODUCTION

In present scenario, computers are common companion of both doctors and nurses in corporate hospitals, and even most of nursing homes. It is also a duty of nursing staff to take care of computers and conduct maintenance tasks to avoid sudden breakdown of computer or loss of data. One cannot afford sudden breakdown of computers or loss of data, which indirectly increases the workload on nursing staff. Also, basic knowledge of maintenance and taking good care of computers will help you to become tech-savvy and utilize this technology to its best advantage.

Few of the maintenance tasks are easy and do not require special training. Other tasks are not difficult, but require initial training and supervision. We can broadly divide maintenance of computer in two categories:

1. Maintenance of hardware.
2. Maintenance of software.

Here are few 'do it yourself tasks', which will help to take care of the personal computer (PC).

MAINTENANCE OF COMPUTER HARDWARE

Clean Your Computer

Two most important enemies of the PCs are the heat and moisture. These cause damage to the device and its electronic circuits. The most common causes of overheating are dust and dirt. Though there is central processing unit (CPU) cooling fan inside the PC, but clogged vent due to dust and dirt, prevents hot air moving out of the case. This causes the cooling fan to run longer and harder, increasing power consumption and chances of fan getting damaged faster. Further, a thin coating of dust or dirt over the components can raise their temperature, thus damaging those components.

If your PC resides in an air conditioned and dust-free environment, one need less frequent cleaning, but in most real world locations, frequent cleaning outside as well as inside the case.

Requirements

Lint-free wipes (a type of cloth used to clean your spectacles), a small blower for compressed air and mild cleaning solution.

Before Cleaning

Turn off and unplug the system.

Cleaning the Case

Wipe the case and then clear ventilation ports to clear obstructions. Compressed air is great for this, but do not blow dust into the PC or to its optical and other drives. Keep all the cables firmly attached to their connectors on the case, to prevent malfunction after finishing the task.

Cleaning the Mouse

Optical mouse has almost replaced traditional mechanical ball mouse. Optical mouse does not require much effort to clean. All you need to do clean the bottom of the mouse without opening the mouse body. Get a soft cloth dipped in water and gently rub it over the soft pads. Once the pads become slightly wet (not soaked), pick a clean white sheet of paper and run the mouse over it. The paper will absorb any of the remaining dust or sticky grease. There are chances that some grease night stuck to the mousepad. Apply some mild cleaning solution to the surface and wipe it with the cloth. Clean the center 'eye' of the mouse with cotton swab or earbud. Make sure to get into the groove of this eye, but do not press too hard or rub on this eye.

Cleaning the Keyboard

Turn the keyboard upside down and shake it to clear the crumbs between the keys. If that does not suffice, use blower. If keys are sticking or the keyboard is really dirty, lift the keys off with the help of two pencils with broken tips, for easier cleaning. Do this task gently; otherwise it will damage the keyboard.

Cleaning the Monitor

Wipe the monitor case and clear its vent of obstructions, without pushing dust into the unit. Clean the screen with a standard glass cleaner and a lint-free cloth.

Cleaning Computer Disk, Digital Versatile Disk and Read Only Memory

Use a good quality lens cleaner computer disk (CD) to clean lenses of your CD/digital versatile disk-read only memory (DVD-ROM). Simply follow the instructions mentioned in product insert. Gently wipe each disk with a moistened, soft cloth. Use a motion that starts at the center of the disk and then moves outward toward the edge. Never wipe a disk in a circular motion.

Cleaning Printer

1. Remove dust with the help of a blower.
2. Clean the exterior with damp cloth.
3. Clean the delicate interior with the help of soft cloth and alcohol.
4. For inkjet printer: Clean the printhead by selecting a program on computer. Go to control panel and select printing preferences. Once you have selected the printer, the computer will guide you through the process of cleaning the printhead. If the printer has self-cleaning option in its menu, choose it and let it do for you.
5. For laser printer: Switch off and disconnect power cable, remove paper trays, eject toner cartridge from printer and put it on newspaper or used paper. Clean the toner cartridge which is inside the machine by wiping the area with soft cloth (clean up any paper shredding and spoiled toner powder). Wipe off the roller.

Note: Never use liquid to clean; instead soak the piece of cloth with liquid to clean the printer.

Check Your Power Protection

Secure the cables plugged into your surge protector. Check the unit's warning indicator, if it has one. Surge protectors may power your PC even after being compromised by a voltage spike (making your system susceptible to a second spike). If your power protector does not have a warning indicator and your area suffers frequent power outages, replace it with one that has such an indicator.

Maintenance Tips

Following are some of the useful and practical tips for the regular maintenance of the computers:

1. Keep the computer off the floor to minimize dust entry.
2. Let the computer breathe easy; do not keep it in a closed space like inside the furniture.
3. Be careful not to knock or drop your computer and do not put any objects on top of it. The case, although strong, is not made to support extra weight.
4. When transporting your computer, put it in a carrying case.
5. Keep your computer away from magnetic fields. Magnetic fields can erase data on hard drives and cause the CPU cooling fan to malfunction.
6. Never turn off your computer when the hard drive light is on because data on the hard drive could be lost or corrupted.
7. Avoid subjecting your computer to extreme temperature changes. As a general rule, your computer is safest at temperatures that are comfortable for you.
8. Keep all liquids and other foods away from your computer.
9. Avoid dusty or dirty work environments.

MAINTENANCE OF COMPUTER SOFTWARE

Defragment Drives

Fragmentations happen to hard disk (HD) overtime as you save, change or delete files. The changes that save to a file, are often stored at a location on the HD that is different from the original file. Additional changes are saved to even more locations. Overtime both the file and the HD itself become fragmented and the computer slows down as it has to look in many different places to open a file. Disk defragmenter is a tool that rearranges the data on HD and reunites fragmented files, so the computer can run more efficiently. In latest versions of Windows, disk defragmenter runs on a schedule, so you do not have to remember to run it although you can still run it manually or change the schedule it uses.

How to Defragment?

Go to the start menu click on 'all programs,' then click on 'accessories' click on 'system tools,' which will have disk defragmenter option. Defragmentation can take long time; especially it is run for the first time. So it is advisable to start this process at the end of a work day, since the process itself can affect a computer's performance.

Clean Files

Regularly delete all trash and temporary files that you no longer need. While in ideal situation, temporary files are deleted when the application closes, but it does not happen many times because of poorly written programs, computer crashes, hanging programs and improper shutdowns leaving unnecessary files in hard drive. These files pile up and start eating up HD space, thus impairing computer performance.

How to Clean Files?

Go to start menu click on 'all programs' then click on 'accessories,' again click on 'system tools' that will have 'disk cleanup' option. Select the drive you want to clean. When it is finished, select the items you no longer want.

Files to be Cleaned

Downloaded program files, temporary internet files, temporary files and recycle bin.

Remove Unwanted Applications

Go to start menu click on 'control panel' then click on 'add or remove programs.' Select the application and click the remove button. This will remove the application.

Caution

Do not do this task without supervision. You may land up removing important application if not aware.

Run an Antivirus Program

Antivirus program is a must for every computer. An up-to-date antivirus program can help to protect the computer from viruses, spyware, malware and other infections, but can be incredibly difficult to remove from computer. It is advisable to protect the computer with an antivirus program many times, as these infections cause irreversible loss, which sometimes is difficult to undo by running such programs later on. If you have configured antivirus program to a scheduled scan regularly, most of your job is done. This feature of antivirus program is background scanning. But manual scans are required when you install antivirus for the first time or when you suspect any threat missed earlier. Scheduled antivirus scans may miss a virus, so it is recommended by many to run manual scan periodically.

Updating your antivirus is very important to protect computers from latest threats. If your computer is connected with internet then it is advisable to keep automatic update on, otherwise you need to update the antivirus every time, which is connected to computer through internet.

Backup Your Computer

Many a time we do not realize how many important files, documents and pictures we have on the HD. Having a computer crash and being unable to recover anything, can be extremely a damaging situation. Make sure that you backup all the data at regular intervals. Back up of data related to patients, should be taken after each session per day.

Caution

Never overwrite old data with recent one, if the fresh data has been corrupted. Also, do not restore data without proper supervision.

Give Rest to Your Computer

It is tempting to let PCs run 24/7, but everything needs to rest occasionally. It is recommended to put your computer to hibernate when not at work. It saves your work and almost powers off, but comes back faster than having to perform a full boot-up. Another less preferred option is to set your PC to sleep, which saves power.

Best option to give rest and healthy life to your computer is to shut down when not in use. Rebooting the computer is another option. Though there is no standard time frame for how long you can keep a PC running without rebooting, but when computer starts giving trouble it is a good idea to reboot, thus giving the machine a fresh start. As you open and close applications, fragments of memory can build, slowing the computer. A reboot frees those memories, thus optimizing the performance.

SCHEDULE OF COMPUTER MAINTENANCE TASKS

Here is the schedule of maintenance tasks for your computer, which would never let you miss any aspect of computer care and help to keep computer healthy.

Daily Tasks

- Virus scan
- Backup (twice or thrice daily, depending on number of sessions).

Monthly Tasks

- Cleaning of case, keyboard, mouse, monitor, printer
- Clean files
- Remove unwanted applications
- Defragmentation.

Yearly Tasks

- Open case and clean
- Test backup battery [complementary metal-oxide-semiconductor (CMOS)]
- Test contacts of adapter cards
- All these three tasks require professional help.

On Failure

Clean CD/DVD-ROM drive (lens cleaning).

CONCLUSION

The maintenance of computer hardware and software are vital components of day to day computer usage. A regular and effective scheduling of these tasks goes to long way in getting the best output from the machine.

FURTHER READING

1. Available from http://daol.aol.com/articles/pc-maintenance/
2. Available from http://pcsupport.about.com/od/maintenance/u/maintain-your-computer.htm [Accessed February 5, 2014].
3. Available from http://support.gateway.com/s/manlib/notebooks/solo1150/8507028/maintain.htm [Accessed February 5, 2014].
4. Available from http://www.abc-computers.com/news-events/blog/pc-maintenance-checklist-5-tips-to-help-you-take-care-of-your-pc/
5. Available from http://www.pcworld.com/article/116583/article.html

5

Backing up the Data

Rajinder Gulati

INTRODUCTION

Data loss is the worst thing to happen. Hence, there is a need to backup the data onto a secure system. Many people are yet unaware of where to store the data safely. Digital data can be stored either locally or remotely. For local storage, a physical backup device such as external hard disk, computer disk (CD), digital video disk (DVD), universal serial bus (USB) flash drive, etc. are required. For saving the data on the remote location, the data is transferred online using the internet, which is also called online backup. Online storage is also referred to as the cloud storage. By definition, cloud storage is a model of networked enterprise storage, where data is stored in virtualized pools of storage, which are generally hosted by third parties. Physically, the resource of cloud storage may span across multiple servers and multiple locations.

EXTERNAL HARD DRIVE OR CLOUD BACKUP

Both options have distinct advantages and disadvantages, so knowing exactly what those are can help to choose the method that is best suited for the data.

External Hard Disk

External USB hard drives are data storage devices used for storing and retrieving digital information using rapidly rotating disks (platters) coated with magnetic material. Continuously improved hard disk drive (HDD) has maintained this position into the modern era of servers and personal computers. An HDD retains its data even when power off. Data is read in a random-access manner, meaning individual blocks of data can be stored or retrieved in any order rather than sequentially. These are less expensive, more reliable and easier to use than ever, which means the market is saturated with dozens of drives to choose from. With a focus on performance, design and functionality, one can choose the best portable hard drive as per his/her needs. Considering the cost-effectiveness, the availability of 500 gigabyte (GB), 1 and 2 terabyte (TB) external hard disks offer a very suitable and convenient option for taking a backup of huge amount of data. Most of the currently available external hard disks offer advanced features in a slim, stylish design that enable the users to save and access their data quickly and conveniently, wherever they go (Fig. 5.1).

Advantages

Cost factor: External hard drives are one time investment, especially when buying a budget external hard drive because you only have to invest once to get full potential. There is no need to sign up for a service that bills you monthly for features that might not need.

Performance: It depends upon the specifications including the storage capacity and transfer speed. The best portable hard drives come in different storage capacities ranging from 500 GB to 2 TB, offering plenty of space for all photos, media and documents. If storage needs increase you can just buy another external hard drive or replace your old one with a model that has more storage. This makes it a very flexible solution. External hard drive can boast about high-data transfer speed, which also depends upon the size of the files being transferred. The USB 3.0 transfer speed has increased dramatically with external hard drives and it does not matter, if you want to backup your high-definition (HD) video collection or a huge photo album.

Security: In case you are very security concerned, external hard drive gives you the flexibility you need to encrypt your files and make them as secure as you want them to be by password protection. Also, you are the only person who has access to your files.

Fig. 5.1: External hard disk

Disadvantages

1. External hard disk might fail or get lost, so one would be without the data.

2. External hard disk needs to be kept connected at all times, which makes it impractical on long run.
3. For non-technical persons who are unable to take care of the encryption, there is always a security risk of data being stolen or viewed by others.

Pen Drive

Being around for last few years, USB pen drives are a popular and an effective devices to store and transfer the data from one device to another. A USB flash drive is a storage device that consists of flash memory with an integrated USB interface. Pen drives are removable and rewritable and physically easily portable. With the steady improvements and low pricing, multiple options have become available with a storage capacity of up to 16 GB have now become easily available. Used carefully these offer multiple write and erase cycles and a long shelf life.

Apart from transferring the data from one computer to another, storage and backup, there are several other uses of the USB flash drive. Some of these drives include backup software for the ease as it makes the backup process automatic. Several other of its benefits include are the encryption of the data, running an alternate operating system and to carry applications that run on the host computers without the necessity of the installations. These can also offer to help the system maintenance, trouble shooting and the recovery of the system or the network.

Cloud Storage Devices Backup

Cloud storage can also be referred to as online space used for storing the data.

Advantages

Unmatched accessibility and flexibility: While an external hard drive limits one to backing up computers, cloud storage allows to backup files stored on any internet-connected device. The best cloud computing services allow to upload and save any type of file you would save on local hard drive from word documents to music files and everything in between. Furthermore, you can access those stored files from any web browser.

Security: Most cloud storage services have encryption technology, which secures your files from third parties. Cloud storage services allow you to select folders and share them with friends and family. Only the people who should have access to your files will get it.

Affordability: Cloud storage has become very cheap in the last couple of years. Service providers have reduced their rates consistently giving you more storage for less money. Many top cloud storage services also offer a limited amount of free storage, anywhere from 2 to 25 GB. This allows you to try the service with no obligation to see if it is a good fit for you and to store a limited number of files that you can access from anywhere.

Disadvantages

Speed variability: Cloud storage transfer speeds can be slow depending on the internet connection and it might take a while until all of your files are transferred to the cloud storage provider. So, if you have terabytes of data that you want to backup and stored in the cloud, you need to be very patient as this can take days together.

Ongoing cost: You need to sign up and pay regularly (monthly or yearly basis), if you want to use the full potential of cloud storage services. Although the cost may be low, it needs consideration before you start using cloud storage facility.

Trust: The service provider of cloud storage facility needs to be trusted as you are transferring your most important files to a service.

Which Backup Option is Best?

The backup method that will work best for largely depends on the type of data you want to store and how to access it. For business and perhaps some consumers, who need to store proprietary or sensitive information, local storage is the most secure option. External hard drives are more cost-effective than cloud services, especially when you store large amounts of data; portable hard drives have a lower cost per gigabyte, so you get more storage capacity.

If convenience and flexibility are priorities, cloud storage will give the unfettered access to data over any internet connection. This is especially important, if routinely use different computers (e.g. a work computer and a personal laptop) or store data on multiple internet-enabled devices.

CONCLUSION

No matter, which method you choose, both cloud storage and external hard drives perform superbly when it comes to effectively backing up and storing the data, but with a word of caution. Using only external hard drives for data storage can be dangerous; hard drives fail or might get stolen, so you will be without the data. The good thing is, should not have to rely on one single backup. It is strongly recommended that one backup the data on an external hard drive, as well as have online backup service as an additional backup layer.

FURTHER READING

1. Available from http://www.cloudstoragereviews.org/cloud-storage-vs-external-hard-drive/ [Accessed September 25, 2014].
2. Available from http://cloud-services-review.toptenreviews.com/
3. Available from http://external-hard-drive-review.toptenreviews.com/external-hard-drive-vs.-cloud-storage-which-is-right-for-your-file-backups-html
4. Available from http://www.onlinebackupreviews.org/online-backup-vs-external-hard-drive/ [Accessed September 30, 2014].

6

Computer Ergonomics

Bakulesh M Chauhan

INTRODUCTION

Ergonomics derives from two Greek words, 'ergon' meaning work and 'nomoi' meaning natural laws, to create a word that means the science of work and a person's relationship to that work. The applied science of equipment design, as for the workplace, intended to maximize productivity by reducing operator fatigue and discomfort.

The International Ergonomics Association has adopted this technical definition—ergonomics is the scientific discipline concerned with the understanding of interactions among humans and other elements of a system and the profession that applies theory, principles, data and methods to design in order to optimize human well-being and overall system performance. That is not the most efficient definition of what ergonomics is. Let us keep things simple. Ergonomics is the science of making things comfortable. It also makes things efficient and when one thinks about it comfortable just another way of making things efficient. However, for simplicity, ergonomics makes things comfortable and efficient.

Ongoing changes in technology, changes in the way one performs, and where and how people work are occurring at a rapid pace. Nowhere is the change more evident than in the use of computers. This new technology has brought on new demands for information as well as new and more sophisticated computing systems. Today, almost every one of us interacts with computers on a daily basis to create new things and ideas, produce documents, correspond with friends and associates and to retrieve information. Along with the expanding use of this technology have come reports about adverse health changes for computer users.

WHAT IS ERGONOMICS?

Ergonomics is the study of how people physically interact with their work for fitting the job, the equipment and the work environment to the worker. It is the application of scientific information concerning humans to the design of objects, systems and environment for human use. Ergonomics comes into everything, which involves people. Work systems, sports and leisure, health and safety should all embody ergonomics principles, if well-designed.

COMPUTER ERGONOMICS

Computers have revolutionized the way one works. People whose occupations involve spending prolonged period of time at a computer workstation are subjected to stresses that may lead to painful, debilitating conditions. The resulting stress may cause higher levels of fatigue and tension during the day. One of the major contributing factors for stress is awkward or non-optimal body positions, which are mainly due to improper work station layout. Computer ergonomics tells us all about it. Further it suggests how best one can use computers without stressing themselves.

Working with a video display terminal (VDT), i.e. computer monitor and a keyboard can be productive, rewarding and a lot of fun. Unfortunately, prolonged postures, coupled with high levels of concentration and the occasional frustration of things going less than perfectly, can lead to physical problems. Basic understanding in the way one person 'interface' with the computer can help prevent common health-related VDT and keyboard problems. A little knowledge of the principles of ergonomics, how people interact safely and efficiently with machines, and with their work environment discomfort, and maximize both productivity and enjoyment.

Nursing is associated with high rates of musculoskeletal disorders from patient handling and nurses are at high risk for developing cumulative trauma disorders, which can result from computer usage. Although, there are many benefits to using computers in the workplace, nurses need to incorporate ergonomic factors into work settings to promote safe workplace environments. Thus, it is important that adequate attention to be paid towards computer ergonomics-related policies and have recommendations about computer workstation design and related research in nursing workplace settings. The idea is to help to computer savvy nurses, to be able to use computer without health problems and sneaking into ruin their fun or decrease their productivity.

Ergonomic Workstation Guidelines

Ergonomic furniture should be designed to facilitate task performance, minimize fatigue and injury by fitting equipment to the body size, strength and range of motion of the user. Office furnishings, which are generally available, have adjustable components that enable the user to modify the workstation to accommodate different physical dimensions and the requirements of job. Ergonomically designed furniture can reduce pain and injury, increase productivity, improve morale and decrease complaints. Design objectives should support humans to achieve the operational objectives for which they are responsible. There are three goals to consider in human-centered design:

1. Enhance human abilities.
2. Overcome human limitations.
3. Foster user acceptance.

To achieve these objectives, there are several key elements of ergonomics to consider, which are as follows:

1. Equipment: Video display terminals.
2. Software design: System and screen design for greater usability.
3. Workstation design: Chairs, work surfaces and accessories.
4. Environment-space planning, use of colors, lighting, acoustics, air quality and thermal factors.
5. Training: Preparing workers to deal with technology.

Machine Set-up

Visibility

When computer work environments are being planned, both overall lighting levels the positioning of lights and windows must be considered. User must be able to see what he/she are doing easily to avoid eye strain and neck pain. Have adequate amounts of light. Fluorescent lights are not very good; the so-called 'natural spectra' fluorescent lights are not quite as bad, incandescent lighting is better and indirect, natural (sun) light is best. Reduce glare as much as possible, not only on the screen, but also on the rest of the work areas including the keyboard. Ways of reducing both direct and indirect glare include the use of light-absorbing blinds or curtains. Hoods, drapes, glare screens and changing the lights can do wonders. Using the control knobs on the monitor; is more helpful. Do not be afraid to fiddle around with the tilt and height positions of the monitor. Rearrange things until it can be seen well and it feels comfortable.

However, paper-based work often requires more light, particularly for poor quality or handwritten text. Elder workers may also require more light. In these cases task lighting (small lamps for a specific area) can be used. Methods used to control light from windows should allow for user control. Roller, vertical or venetian blinds or thick curtains can be used. However, care should be taken in the selection and sizing of coverings to ensure that the light is fully blocked.

Where possible, terminals should be positioned such that the operator's line of sight is parallel to windows and overhead fluorescent lights (Fig. 6.1). Workstations should be located between rows of overhead lights.

Antiglare screens should be used only after other methods have proved unsuccessful. Although, these reduce indirect glare from the screen, the mesh types also tend to attract dust and some glass models create more reflections. This may increase visual demands on the operator.

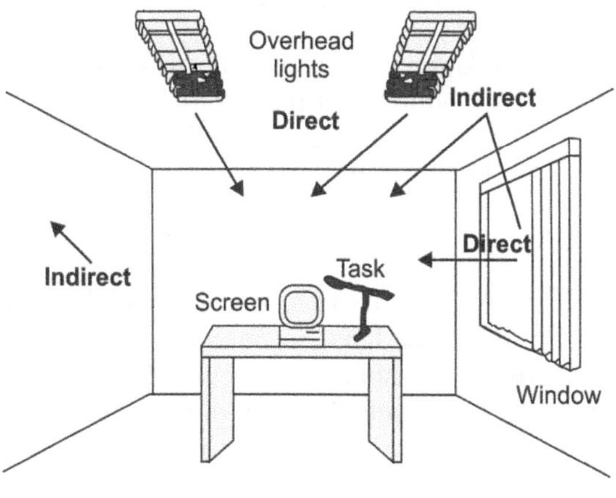

Fig. 6.1: Proper lighting for workstation

Chairs

As with visibility factors, experiment with chair height and/or tilt. Try different chairs. Keep trying until it gets the way body likes.

Seat height: It should be pneumatically adjusted, while seated. A range of 40–52 cm of the floor should accommodate most users. Thighs should be horizontal, lower legs vertical, feet flat on the floor or on a footrest. Seat height should also allow a 90° angle at the elbows for typing.

Seat width and depth: A seat width of 43–51 cm suffices for most people and should be deep enough to permit the back to contact the lumbar backrest without cutting into the backs of knees. The front edge should be rounded and padded. The seat slant should be adjustable (0°–10°). Avoid bucket-type seats. The seat should swivel easily.

Backrest: The backrest should offer firm support, especially in the lumbar (lower back) region, should be 20–48 cm wide and should be easily adjustable both in angle and height, while sitting. The optimum angle between seat and back should permit a working posture of at least 90° between the spine and thighs. Seat pan angle and backrest height and angle should be coordinated to allow for the most comfortable weight load on the spinal column.

Seat material: A chair seat and back should be padded enough to allow comfortable circulation. If a seat is too soft, the muscles must always adjust to maintain a steady posture, causing strain and fatigue. The seat fabric should 'breathe' to allow air circulation through clothes to the skin.

Armrests: These are optional, depending on user preference and task performed. They should not restrict movement or impede the worker's ability to get close enough to the work surface. The worker should not rest his/her forearms, while typing.

Keyboards

Be sure to get the right height to prevent too much bend at the wrist and allow the forearm to have some support. The arms should hang loose to prevent the shoulder muscles from cramping. Many keyboards can tilt; unfortunately, most of them tilt the wrong way. Tilt the keyboard to help the wrist stay straight, that is raise the space bar end and lowering the 'top' (the F1, F2, etc.) end. Tilting the keyboard the other way, (space bar lower and 'top' row higher) can predispose to carpal tunnel syndrome.

When working at a keyboard, the operator should be sitting with the upper arms hanging naturally from the shoulders. The elbows should be bent at roughly a 90° angle, when the fingers are in typing position on the home row of the keyboard. This posture allows the arms and wrists to be held in a natural and relaxed position that puts the least amount of physical stress on muscles and joints.

Mouse

The continual clicking and small precise motions involved in mouse use are a repetitive action that can be a health hazard. A few basic rules can be helpful in handling convenient mouse. Input device safer and more comfortable:

1. Hold the mouse loosely. 'White knuckling' the mouse creates too much tension. Use a light touch, while clicking.
2. Use whole arm and shoulder to move the mouse, not just the wrist. Do not rest forearm on the desk, while moving the mouse.
3. Do not lift little finger (pinkie), use all of fingers to lightly hold the mouse.
4. Keep wrist relaxed and neutral, not bent. The click button should be about the same height as keyboard.
5. Avoid prolonged postures. Rotate shoulders; gently shake hands and fingers four or five times per hour.
6. Left handers should use a 'left-handed' mouse or configure the mouse to work best with their different (mirror image) hand shape.

Desks

The best way to provide the proper screen and keyboard heights for all operators is to use split-level tables or desks that allow each height to be adjusted independently. This allows for proper work postures for a range of user sizes. However, a fixed desk of suitable height, the correct use of an adjustable chair and a footrest and/or monitor stand where necessary, will also allow for suitable postures.

Make enough space, so that one has room to work, especially in case of moving the mouse around. Use a paper holder to keep letters or books semivertical and at eye level. The work space should be set up, so that one need not twist the neck. Documents should be positioned at the same height and next to the VDT, especially if a lot of time is to be spent at these tasks. Make the work space user friendly.

Keep the eyes in distance, while working with VDT. Electromagnetic radiations follows the inverse square rule, which is to say the further away one is from the source, the weaker they get and they do so quickly. One can protect themself with space. It is recommend to stay at least 75 cm (30 inches) away from terminal and at least 1 m (40 inches) from other terminals.

Keep it fixed. X-ray and other radiation production increases dramatically, when the VDT is damaged, improperly maintained or just plain worn out.

Any table, desk or stand used for computer work must be deep enough for both the keyboard and the monitor to be in front of the worker. In cases where space is limited, the use of flat screens is one option for freeing up space. There should be sufficient leg-room.

Document Holders

Computer work often involves entering information from source documents. These should be located beside the screen and in the same plane. This reduces the size and amount of head and eye movements between the document and the screen, and decreases the likelihood of muscular and visual fatigue. The best way to position documents correctly is to use an adjustable document holder. These are usually mounted on a flexible arm that is fixed to a base or clamps to the edge of the desk. The clamping type is preferable, if desk space is limited. Before purchasing a holder, consider the size and thickness of the documents to be used and choose a holder that will accommodate them. A slant board is one option for supporting larger document.

Telephone Work

Increasingly, workers are required to use a keyboard, while on the telephone. This often results in awkward head, neck and back postures with the receiver cradled between the shoulder and head to leave both hands free. Workers require to use a computer, while on the telephone for long periods tend to experience discomfort, particularly in the head and back. In such cases, headsets should be used. Hands-free phones are also an option, where the office space and task are appropriate. A spacer or cradle that mounts to the handset is not a preferred option. Although, it improves the head position, a static effort is still needed to hold the handset in place.

Human Set-up

Posture

One posture is not perfect. One do not have to be 'military' but getting comfortable is essential. Footrests help (or a book or lunchpail or anything handy to rest your feet up a bit) as do cushions if chair is not providing adequate support. The most important rule is to avoid prolonged positions. Shake hands and shoulders now and then. Keep loose.

Eyes

After good lighting and avoiding glare, the most important eye consideration is to look away from the screen occasionally. It really helps. Also, do not forget to blink. Blinking moistens the eyes to prevent burning from dryness.

Warm up

Just as an athlete prepares for the game by stretching and loosening the joints and muscles to prevent injury and enhance performance, should one also prepare for a marathon session surfing the internet. Some shoulder rolls, neck stretches, wrist wiggles and leg stretches should be done before logging in. Prevention is better than cure.

Breaks

If you hold any part of you in one position for longer than an hour, you set yourself up for stiff joints, achy muscles, tendon fatigue and ligament weakness; not to mention decreased efficiency and diminished concentration. If you are focused on what you are doing, you can lose track of time unless you purposely schedule breaks. Have the computer clock on screen or set the alarm on your watch or somehow let yourself know about the passage of time. Then, at least once in an hour, (every ½ an hour would be better), get right up off your seat and walk around, stretch, yawn, wiggle, breath, get the blood flowing and stimulate the joints. It is worth the time and trouble as you will feel better, work sharper and get more done. Take advantage of unscheduled 'downtime'. Instead of staring at the little hourglass and wishing it would go faster, do something beneficial for body.

If you already have mechanical body problems such as neck arthritis or carpal tunnel syndrome, it is necessary to take breaks more frequently; on the order of three or four mini breaks per hour. Preventing a flair-up is far superior to irritating these disorders.

Proper Setup of Equipment

Goal: With the appropriate furniture adjustments and ergonomic equipment, VDT workstation should accommodate the proper body postures as illustrated below (Fig. 6.2).

Seating: Adjust the height of the seat to allow for:

- Feet to plant comfortably on the floor (or footrest)
- Knees to bend at 90° or slightly greater
- Thighs to rest parallel to the floor.
  Adjust seatback position to allow for:
- Hips to bend at 90° or slightly greater
- Adequate low back support
- Adjust seat pan depth to allow for a 5–10 cm gap between the front edge of seat and back of knees.

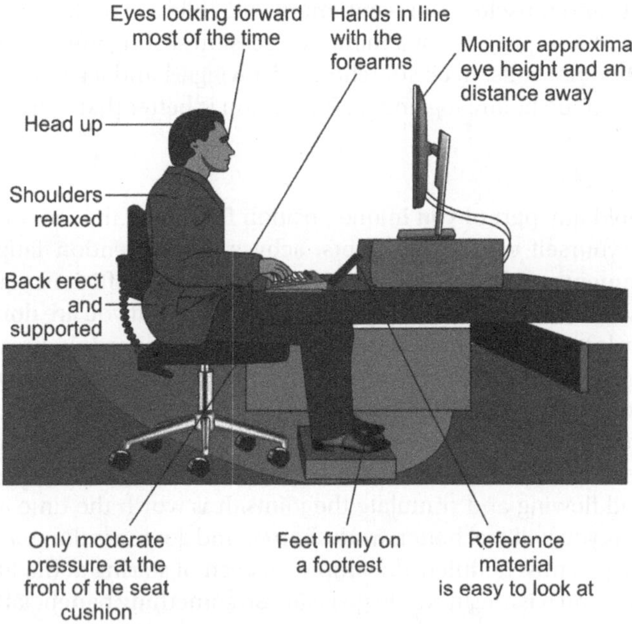

Fig. 6.2: Proper posture for workstation

Mouse and Keyboard Height

Adjust mouse and keyboard height to allow for:
- Hands at elbow height or slightly lower
- Forearms and hands to form straight lines
- Shoulders to be relaxed, with elbows hanging close to the sides.

Monitor Placement

Adjust your monitor position to allow for:
- The top of the screen to align at or slightly below eye level
- Straight-forward monitor viewing
- A comfortable distance between 40 and 52 cm
- An upright head posture with chin tucked in.

Relaxing Exercises

To help relieve office stress from body, try incorporating several of these stretching exercises in the morning warm-up and daytime work schedule. While performing these stretches the following should be considered.

Do Not's

- Bounce or use jerky motions
- Stretch till it hurts.

Do's

- Breathe deeply and relax
- Extend the stretch until it's comfortable
- Move smoothly and slowly.

Caution: In case of any injury or any type of reoccurring discomforts, immediately report about injury/symptoms and obtain a medical evaluation. These stretching exercises are not provided to cure any existing problems, but may help in preventing any future ones. Individuals with previous injury should consult with personal physician before performing these exercises on a routine basis.

Eyes

Close eyes tightly for a second, then open them widely (repeat several times). Refocus eyes momentarily on an object at least 20 feet away.

Hands

Spread fingers wide apart and hold for 10 seconds, form fists for 10 seconds (repeat several times). Place hands together with fingers spread apart and fingertips at chin level. Slowly lower hands, peel them apart and reverse the process. Repeat several times.

Neck

Slowly turn head to side and hold for 10 seconds. Alternate sides and repeat several times. Slowly, tilt head to side and hold for 5–10 seconds. Alternate sides and repeat several times.

Shoulders

Slowly shrug shoulders in a forward circular motion. Alternate to reverse circular motion.

Low back

With hands on hips and feet about shoulder width apart, slowly lean hips forward and shoulders slightly back. Hold the stretch for 5–10 seconds.

LAPTOP ERGONOMICS

Laptops are a wonderful technological tool that can increase productivity and creativity. They allow to take immense computing power with one where ever required. Unfortunately, certain ergonomics features are compromised for the sake of portability. Posture, keyboard spacing, screen size and positioning and pointing devices usually take the biggest ergonomic hit.

Even though laptops are designed for portability, many people use them as a desktop computer. Despite the poor ergonomics inherent in most laptops, certain steps can be taken to create a sound ergonomic laptop setup as a desktop. Whether it is as a main computer or a temporary setup, he/she can improve their ergonomics. Use of laptop computers does present the potential for significant health concerns, however, as laptops do not provide proper ergonomic positioning for the user.

Ergonomic Issues with Laptops

1. **Keyboard spacing:** Laptop keyboards are often compact with odd placement of some keys and cramped spacing of others. Hand cramps and repetitive stress injuries to wrists are more of a concern on compact keyboards.
2. **Monitor size:** Laptop screens are often smaller than desktop monitors. Small screens can cause more eye strain than larger ones. The screen is too close to the user, which causes eye strain.
3. **Monitor placement:** The relation of the keyboard to monitor on a laptop is fixed. This either causes neck strain (when the laptop is placed low enough to allow for reasonably good wrist/arm positioning) or excessive wrist/arm strain (when the laptop is placed so that the screen is at eye level to prevent neck strain).
4. **Small pointers:** Laptops usually have an integrated pointing device such as a touch pad or dot. These devices are adequate for their task, but not very comfortable or easy to use for long periods of time. Wrist-related repetitive stress injuries pop up here as well.

All of these problems can be remedied at a very reasonable cost. From an ergonomic standpoint, laptops are designed only for occasional use (e.g. occasional weekends, while traveling, for classroom presentations, etc.). Laptops are not ideal for extended periods of use; however, they are increasingly used in this manner.

If the laptop will serve as the user's primary computer or used frequently or for extended periods then the following items should also be provided with each laptop computer:

1. For general use, place the laptop on a flat surface with the screen tilted back 110°–150°.
2. A separate, full-sized keyboard and pointing device. Most laptops these days are already equipped with a port for a separate keyboard and mouse.
3. A monitor riser to raise the monitor screen to eye level. There are many types of risers available at many different price ranges. A simple and effective riser can be made by stacking books under the laptop computer until the appropriate height is achieved.
4. A 'docking station' is the best ergonomic laptop solution. These devices allow to plug in laptop to a base station that has a monitor, keyboard and mouse already connected. Basically there is a desktop setup with a removable computer that just happens to have a keyboard and screen attached.

5. If there is no access to a docking station, the next best option is to place the laptop on a laptop stand and use an external keyboard and mouse. If one cannot use a stand even books can be used under the laptop.
6. If not already owned, additional equipment (e.g. ergonomic chair, desk, keyboard tray, etc.) may be necessary to allow users to position their bodies properly (i.e. forearms and hands parallel or lower to the floor, thighs parallel or higher to the floor, monitor at eye level). Please note that many slide-out trays provided with modular office furniture do not offer proper ergonomic placement of the arms and are often too short to allow the pointing device (mouse/trackball) to be on the same level as the keyboard.

Some Good Practices

1. Maintain a comfortable viewing distance (in the range of 40-74 cm). Font size can be adjusted to allow the laptop to be placed for both good viewing and a comfortable body position.
2. Place laptop to minimize glare from lights and windows.
3. Adjust brightness and contrast to suit lighting conditions.
4. Keep screen clean.
5. Have regular eye examinations and inform the ophthalmologist about the computer usage.

Carrying the Laptop

1. When carrying the laptop over any distance, shift the load from side-to-side and between hands and shoulders.
2. Batteries add weight. Avoid carrying an extra battery if there is access to alternating current (AC) or power.
3. Avoid putting a lot of extra materials into laptop case. Use another brief case, if needed. This will reduce the load on one side and better balance the overall load.
4. Avoid carrying a lot of hard copies of documents in the computer case. Work from electronic copies where possible.
5. If carrying more than one item, try to balance the load on both sides of the body.
6. Consider using a cart to reduce the amount of carrying.
7. Backpacks are a good alternative when carrying over uneven terrain or in snowy conditions.

RECOMMENDATIONS

Workstation Layout

1. The monitor should be set at a height, so that the neck will be straight.
2. Elbow joints should be at about 90° with the arms hanging naturally at the sides.
3. Keep hands in line with the forearms, so the wrists are straight, not bending up, down or to either side.
4. Thighs should be roughly parallel to the floor, with feet flat on the floor or footrest.
5. If necessary, use a footrest to support your feet.
6. Chair should be fully adjustable (i.e. for seat height, backrest height and seat pan tilt and preferably, armrests). It should have a well-formed lumbar (lower back) support to help maintain the lumbar curve.
7. There should be enough space to use the mouse. Use a wrist rest or armrest, so that wrist is straight and arm muscles are not overworked.
8. Use an adjustable document holder to hold source documents at the same height, angle and distance as the monitor.

Bifocals, Trifocals and Single-focus Glasses

A computer operator, who wears bifocals, may tilt the head back to view the monitor through the bottom, close vision and part of the glasses. If bifocals cause discomfort or awkward head positions, several approaches can be taken. The screen should be lowered such that the head is in a neutral position while viewing the top line of text or other material.

Alternatively, one could wear single-focus glasses designed specifically for computer work, with the focal distance chosen for viewing distance between the worker and the screen. In this case, it is important that a document holder is also used, to position documents at the same viewing distance. Other options are graduated bifocals, which have no sharp line between the two parts of the lens, trifocals or the use of reverse bifocal lenses, where the computer screen prescription is in the upper part of the lens. Computer users should have their eyes checked regularly and discuss their computer use with their optometrists.

Seating

An office chair should have:

1. A five-prong base, with its feet set in a circle at least as big as the seat itself.
2. Seat height adjustable from 42–51 cm (standard) to 38–45 cm (low height).
3. A covering made with a breathable material and dense foam that gives way no more than 2.5 cm.
4. A seat pan that:
   a. Is large enough to provide support for thighs and buttocks, but not so long that the front edge presses into the backs of the operator's lower legs:
      - Small: 38–42 cm
      - Medium: 42–46 cm
      - Large: Greater than 46 cm.

   b. Has a 'waterfall' front edge (i.e. rounded, downward-curving) to reduce pressure on the underside of the thighs.
   c. Is adjustable, so that it can tilt from 3° forward (i.e. with the front edge 3° down from the horizontal) to 4° back.
   d. Has a width of greater and equal to 45 cm.
5. Backrest that:
   a. With lumbar support adjustable to 15–25 cm above the seat. If the backrest is fixed (a less desirable option) the lumbar support should be within this range.
   b. With the upper edge at a height of 45–55 cm above the seat pan for a standard back. A high back should be greater and equal to 7.5 cm higher than a standard back.
   c. Adjustable angle within a range of 93°–103°. A fixed backrest should be in the range of 93°–103°.
6. Armrests:
   a. Armrest height is adjustable to 19–24 cm or fixed within same range.
   b. Of length greater and equal to 18 cm, but set back at least 15 cm from the edge of the seat.
   c. Should not impede computer work or positioning of chair.
   d. With a distance between armrests of at least 45 cm (or adjustable).

Footrests, where they are necessary, should have a stable surface and be large enough to accommodate both feet easily. The footrest angle could be adjustable, though a fixed footrest is suitable, if it allows for comfortable ankle angles (roughly 90° between foot and leg). Generally, fixed footrest angles are in the range of 0°–30°. Make sure that workers are aware of the importance of adjusting their chairs correctly and know how to make adjustments themselves. Chairs should be readjusted when workers change the height, they will be working for any length of time. For example, from keyboarding to writing.

How to Protect 'Yourself from Strain and Pain'?

Modify body mechanics as follows:

- Do you wear eyeglasses? Make sure they fit properly to avoid tilting your head
- Type with light strokes and try to keep muscles relaxed
- Sit 'tall' aligning ears, shoulders and hips; while sitting, think about making the chair an inch taller
- Switch hands when using a mouse, if you are able
- Completely rest your wrists during breaks, including taking your hands off the mouse.

Adjust work patterns:

- Reduce prolonged computer time whenever possible
- Break work into smaller segments and switch between tasks that use different motions. For example, alternate use of mouse with reading and searching the website.

Move: Movement has many benefits. It relaxes tissues, lubricates joints and prevents stiffness, improves circulation, reduces fatigue and builds stamina. One study showed that heavy computer users, who successfully avoided computer-related pain, moved every 7 minutes. At least every 10 minutes, take a short (10–20 second) break. Take hands off the keyboard and move. In every 30-60 minutes, take a brief (2–5 minute) break to stretch and/or walk around.

Exercise at Your Computer

1. **Neck/Shoulders exercise:**

Neck rotation: Slowly rotate head as far as comfortable to the right, then left.

Shoulder rotation: Rotate shoulders, then reverse directions.

Head side-to-side: Bend the neck, so left ear approaches left shoulder, then repeat for right. Add a little resistance by pressing your hand against the side of the head.

Chin tuck: Slide chin inward, without bending your neck up or down. This is easiest to practice initially against a wall. Tuck chin in, attempting to touch back of neck to the wall, while also maintaining head contact. Do not jam chin down to chest.

Shoulder blade retraction: Pull shoulders down and back.

Shrug: Slowly raise shoulders toward ears and hold for a few seconds. Gradually, bring shoulders down and relax.

2. **Back:**

Shoulder squeeze: Raise your arms in front of body, with elbows bent and thumbs up. Pull elbows back, squeezing shoulder blades together. Hold for a few seconds then release.

Stretch up: Sit up straight and imagine a cable attached to the top of head. Gradually, stretch to be as tall as possible, hold for a few seconds and then relax.

3. **Arms:**

Arm relaxation: Drop the arms and hands to the sides. Gently shake them for a few seconds.

Arm rotation: Raise the arms in front of body. Rotate arms, so palms face up, then rotate so backs of hands face each other.

4. **Hands/Wrists:**

Wrist flex: With elbows on desk, gently use left hand to bend right hand back toward forearm. Hold for a few seconds, then relax. Repeat on other side.

Finger fan: Spread the fingers as far apart as possible, hold, then clench fists, then release.

5. **Feet:**

Toe curl: Flex toes up, then curl toes under; release.

Foot rotation: Circle foot slowly from the ankle, then reverse.

6. **Eyes:**

Eye rolls: Roll the eyes clockwise then counterclockwise briefly.

Palm eyes: Without touching eyes, cup hands lightly over eyes for 30 seconds to rest them from light.

Look away: Exercise your eyes by periodically looking away from your computer to focus on distant objects.

7. **Keep fit:**

Physical fitness can help you avoid and treat problems related to computer use. Build your stamina with exercises for strength, flexibility, and cardiovascular health.

When to Seek Medical Care?

Consult clinician if experienced a persistent or troubling complaint such as constant pain, numbness of a limb or weakness or any other problems that tend to interfere with the daily tasks.

CONCLUSION

Computer ergonomics form an essential tool in the use of personal computers and if one has to avoid all the aches, pains and stress related with the use of these gadgets simple exercises, appropriate posture and well-designed workstation dynamics would go a long way in optimizing their use.

FURTHER READING

1. Ergonomics. Available from URL http://www.apple.com/about/ergonomics/ [Accessed September 2014].
2. Safety and Health. Available from URL http://www.safety.uwa.edu.au/ [Accessed September 2014].
3. Computer Ergonomics; How to Protect Yourself from Strain and Pain. Available from URL http://www.uhs.umich.edu/computerergonomics/ [Accessed September 2014].

7

Microsoft Word, Excel and Access

Nikita Thakkar, Upant Rao Dongre

MICROSOFT WORD

Microsoft word application software program is used to prepare attractive and well-designed or formatted documents. MS-Word is used to prepare business and commercial letters. Mailing list, mail merge, reports can be prepared by word. Word processor has many advantages over typewriter. The attractive document created by word processor can be saved in computer and when required, they can be used again. Spelling and grammar checking is possible, new paragraphs or sentences can be added anywhere in document. The auto page numbering, headers, footers and many other facilities are available with word processing. Due to this retyping is not required and documents can be saved on hard disk.

In Microsoft word, multiple options are available. The appearance and design of document can be changed very quickly by using this options. The font, color and style can be selected to have good appearance and enhance visibility. The page numbers, headers and footers can be used to create attractive document. Tables can be inserted. Formatting tools are provided. The preview option gives clear idea about printout before printing document.

Advantages

1. The user should be not bother for right margin.
2. User should not press enter key for new line unless it is new paragraph or required.
3. **Spelling checker:** Spelling checker tool is provided on tool bar or it can be selected from menu bar to correct the incorrect spellings. When the typing of document is over, user can use this facility of word processor to select spelling checker tool. Each word in document is compared with the software's internal

dictionary. For suspected misspelling, computer displays list of suggested words, in dialogue box.

4. **Search (Find and replace):** The search or find command, looks for every occurrence of a word or sequence of characters. Along with find, user can give replace command to change the word in whole document at once.
5. **Hyper links or hyper text links:** It is a special feature of word processing software. It establishes cross references between different pages of a document or between different files. The other file may be located at some other computer in the network or on internet. The hypertext links are useful to give information of a topic in the different chapters of e-book (electronic book or book on electronic media). The cross reference is established by appropriate tool provided by word processing software.

Disadvantages

1. Microsoft word or MS-Word has the capability to be used as a web publishing program. However, there are significant drawbacks to using **Word** as opposed to a program designed for the job, such as Macromedia Dreamweaver. Microsoft Word produces bloated code, with some code only supported by Internet Explorer browsers.
2. There is no provision for alternate text for users who block images or for users with limited visibility. Image files for Microsoft Word are assigned generic names and may be duplicated on the web page.
3. With the release of Microsoft Office Suite 2007, including Microsoft Word 2007, users of older versions of the software found themselves unable to open, let alone edit, documents received in the later version. The default extension for Microsoft Word 2007 documents is .docx; the default extension for documents in earlier versions of Microsoft Word is .doc.
4. An extra step is necessary to save a version of Microsoft Word 2007 documents in a format compatible with older versions of word.
5. Also, users of the newer version of the software sometimes encounter formatting problems in opening documents created in older versions of Word.

Shortcut Keys

Shortcut	Description
Ctrl + 0	Toggles 6 pts of spacing before a paragraph
Ctrl + A	Select all contents of the page
Ctrl + B	Bold highlighted selection
Ctrl + C	Copy selected text
Ctrl + V	Paste the selected text
Ctrl + D	Open the font preferences window
Ctrl + E	Aligns the line or selected text to the center of the screen
Ctrl + F	Open find box
Ctrl + I	Italic highlighted selection

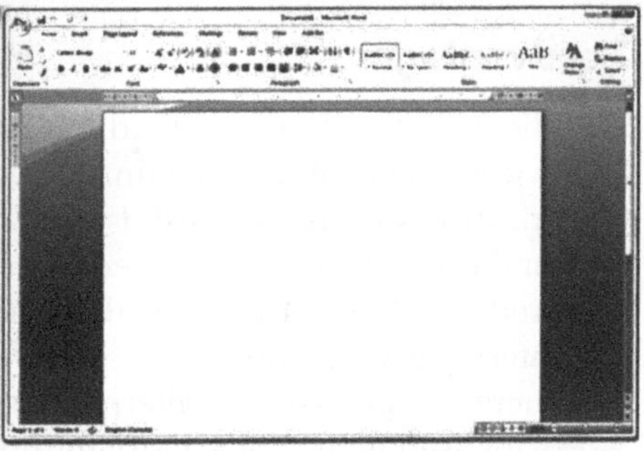

MICROSOFT EXCEL

Workbook: Microsoft Excel is a spreadsheet software program to create files with extension 'xls'. This files are named as 'workbook' as default name. User can rename these files by a meaningful name. When Excel Program starts, worksheet is opened like grid of rows and columns. It consists three sheets indicated by 3 tabs on sheet tab bar. It is just above status bar. By default, 3 sheets viz. sheet-1, sheet-2, and sheet-3 are available in a workbook. The names of sheets can be renamed again if required Excel can provide up to 256 sheets in one workbook.

Different parts of worksheet: A worksheet is a rectangular grid of rows and columns. The rows, columns and cells are the basic elements of worksheet.

Rows and columns: The 65,536 rows are numbered from top to bottom on the left side. The 256 columns are labelled from left to right with letters. The first column is A, then second B and 26th is Z. After this, columns are labelled as AA, AB..... through IV.

Advantages

1. Easy and effective comparisons
2. Powerful analysis of large amounts of data
3. Working together
4. Microsoft Excel Mobile and iPad Apps

Disadvantages

1. One disadvantage of Microsoft Excel is that users cannot enter numbers starting with '0' unless the field of the cell is changed from a number to text.
2. Macros and other mini programs written into Microsoft Excel spreadsheets are prone to virus infections.
3. When a data file is too large, it can make the Excel program run very slowly, especially if all of the data is on one file.

Shortcut Keys

Shortcut	Description
F2	Edit the selected cell
F3	After a name has been created, F3 will paste names
F4	Repeat last action. For example, if you changed the color of text in another cell, pressing F4 will change the text in cell to the same color
F5	Go to a specific cell. For example, C6
F7	Spell check selected text or document

PICTORIAL PRESENTATION

In this topic you will be introduced to pictorial presentation such as charts and graphs. Location and shape of a quantitative distribution can easily be visualized through pictorial presentation such as histogram or frequency polygon.

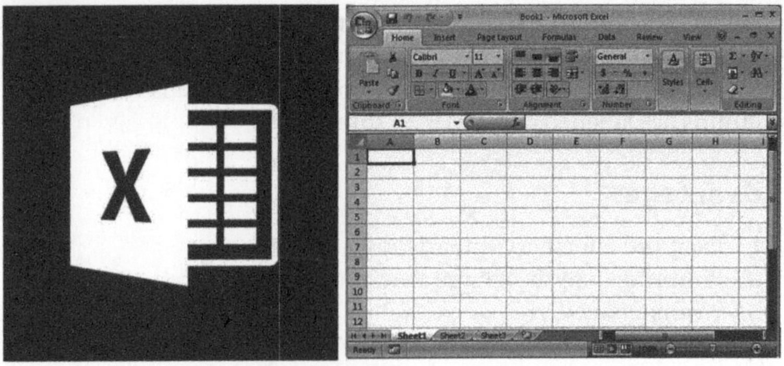

For qualitative data, proportion of any categorical value can be demonstrated by pie chart or bar chart. Comparison of any categorical value between two set of data can be visualized via multiple bar chart.

Thus, pictorial presentation can be very useful in demonstrating some properties and characteristics of a given data distribution. Several pictorials to be discussed are bar chart, multiple bar chart, pie chart, histogram, frequency polygon and cumulative frequency polygon. Statistical package such as Microsoft Excel can be used to draw the above pictorials.

Advantages

1. **Acceptability:** Such report is acceptable to the busy persons because it easily highlights about the theme of the report. This helps to avoid wastage of time.
2. **Comparative analysis:** Information can be compared in terms of graphical representation. Such comparative analysis helps for quick understanding and attention.
3. **Less cost:** Information if descriptive involves huge time to present properly. It involves more money to print the information but graphical presentation can be made in short but catchy view to make the report understandable. It obviously involves less cost.
4. **Decision-making:** Business executives can view the graphs at a glance and can make decision very quickly which is hardly possible through descriptive report.
5. **Logical ideas:** If tables, design and graphs are used to represent information then a logical sequence is created to clear the idea of the audience.

Disadvantages

1. **Costly:** Graphical representation of reports are costly because it involves images, colors and paints. Combination of material with human efforts makes the graphical presentation expensive.
2. **More time:** Normal report involves less time to represent but graphical representation involves more time as it requires graphs and figures which are dependent to more time.
3. **Errors and mistakes:** Since graphical representations are complex, there is each and every chance of errors and mistake. This causes problems for better understanding to general people.
4. **Lack of secrecy:** Graphical representation makes full presentation of information which may hamper the objective to keep something secret.
5. **Problems to select the suitable method:** Information can be presented through various graphical methods and ways. Which should be the suitable method is very hard to select.
6. **Problem of understanding:** All may not be able to get the meaning of graphical representation because it involves various technical matters which are complex to general people.

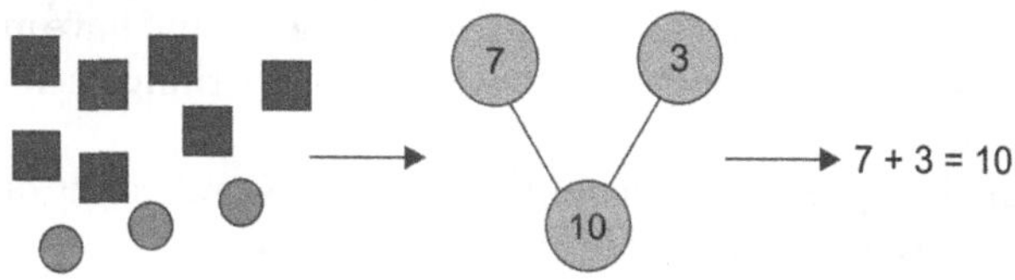

MICROSOFT ACCESS

Microsoft Access is a database management system (DBMS) from Microsoft that combines the relational Microsoft Jet Database Engine with a graphical user interface and software-development tools. It is a member of the Microsoft Office suite of applications, included in the professional and higher editions or sold separately.

Microsoft Access stores data in its own format based on the Access Jet Database Engine. It can also import or link directly to data stored in other applications and databases.

Advantages

1. In addition to using its own database storage file, Microsoft Access also may be used as the 'front-end' of a program while

other products act as the 'back-end' tables, such as Microsoft SQL Server and non-Microsoft products such as Oracle and Sybase.

2. Multiple backend sources can be used by a Microsoft Access Jet Database (ACCDB and MDB formats).
3. Similarly, some applications such as Visual Basic, ASP.NET, or Visual Studio .NET will use the Microsoft Access database format for its tables and queries.
4. Microsoft Access may also be part of a more complex solution, where it may be integrated with other technologies such as Microsoft Excel, Microsoft Outlook, Microsoft Word, Microsoft PowerPoint and ActiveX controls.
5. Access tables support a variety of standard field types, indices, and referential integrity including cascading updates and deletes.
6. Access also includes a query interface, forms to display and enter data, and reports for printing. The underlying Jet database, which contains these objects, is multi-user and handles record-locking.
7. Repetitive tasks can be automated through macros with point-and-click options.
8. It is also easy to place a database on a network and have multiple users share and update data without overwriting each other's work.
9. Data is locked at the record level which is significantly different from Excel which locks the entire spreadsheet.

Disadvantages

1. Microsoft Access is useful for individual departments or small-to-medium business sectors. Any sector whose usage goes beyond 2 GB will hit a wall and discover limitations.
2. All the information from your database is saved into one file. This limits options and how you choose utilize data; slowing down reports, queries, and forms. Its performance becomes slow as the user scales data size. Multimedia data can use up MS Access limited space quickly.
3. It is difficult to publish files a part from static files.
4. Technical limit is 255 concurrent users, but real world limit is 10 to 80 (depending on type of application).

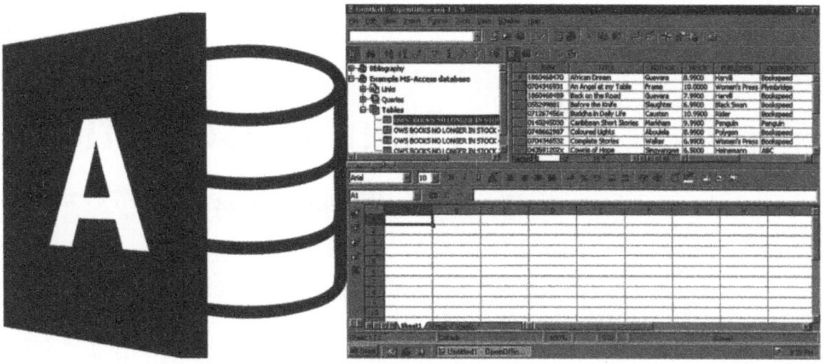

FURTHER READING

1. Wikipedia, https://en.wikipedia.org/wiki/Microsoft_Office

8

PowerPoint Presentation

Neelkamal Kapoor, Pradeep Kapoor

INTRODUCTION

Audio visual (AV) presentations play an important part in scientific and medical gatherings, and are an extremely powerful communication tools in the present times. The use of a visual aid is imperative to enhance the grasp and effect of the message to the target audience. If one can combine text, graphic and animation in a slideshow format to create an illustrative, easy to handle presentation then this goal is well-achieved. The method to achieve this objective is to prepare a PowerPoint presentation. Microsoft PowerPoint is a proprietary commercial presentation program developed by Microsoft and was launched in 1990. It has evolved much since then.

While a properly prepared visual presentation enhances the range, speed, content and the depth of the presentation, in contrast a poorly designed one can fail to deliver the effective messages and resultantly kill the rapport of the speaker with the audience. The following section provides useful and practical tips for creating a clear and effective presentation in meetings, whether they are for scientific purposes or for parent teacher meetings, or for other health education purposes.

USES OF POWERPOINT PRESENTATION

PowerPoint offers following facilities for the AV presentation:

1. Can be hooked to a liquid-crystal display (LCD) projector and an on-screen presentation can be made.
2. Printouts (usually six slides per page for good readability) can be taken, which can be used as handouts.
3. Speakers can print one slide to a page and note down his/her thoughts, which can be consulted while delivering the presentation (speaking notes).
4. Last minute changes and additions are very easily possible.

BEFORE YOU BEGIN

Scientific presentations concern about everything including the purpose of the presentation, defining the things that the audience should know and finally the preparation of the presentation (designing, editing and refining), which is an effective communication with the audience.

Few Facts to Remember Before Making a PowerPoint Presentation

1. Clearly identify the target audience. It is good idea to give a thought about what the audience is going to be like. Whether it is group of students or young parents, or paramedical health workers or doctors, this can help you to decide how to prepare and design the presentation.
2. Write down the thoughts/messages/text, etc. either on paper or on the computer in Microsoft (MS) word program. The scientific content of the presentation is also equally important and must be kept as simple, and easy to follow as much as possible.
3. Enquire precisely about time allotted for the presentation and calculate the desired length of presentation. A seasoned speaker takes, on an average, one minute per slide, for display and explanation. Putting a too much number of slides for your presentation is going to compromise the quality of your presentation and often may fail to convey the message that the speaker would have, otherwise conveyed to the audience.
4. Correlate the text with the grasping capability of the target audience and time allotted, and add/subtract/edit material accordingly.
5. Separate this information for different slides. Each slide should preferably show one idea or aspect of the topic of presentation. Such as, if the speaker wants to show the drug treatment of fever in children, this should appear under the management section of the presentation and be limited to a few slides in a proper sequential order.
6. Rule of six is important for planning a slide, i.e. not more than six lines per slide and six words per line. The idea is try to be as concise and simple as possible.
7. Remember, PowerPoint slide is not only for reading out to the audience but also to put a brief outline, which you can detail in

your talk. The text in the slide should be made in the manner of the phrase and with minimum words allowing the speaker to take the help of the slide in effectively communicating and explaining without reading the entire content shown on the slide. The slides that you show should be your aid in the presentation and not become the whole content by themselves.

MAKING THE SLIDES

1. Select the program of MS PowerPoint in the MS Office.
2. Another menu will open. Point to MS PowerPoint and click to open the program. Sometimes you do not need to go through these steps, if the icon of PowerPoint is given on computer screen itself. In that case one needs to click on the icon directly.
3. A screen would be open to displaying various options including one for creating a new PowerPoint presentation.
4. Select (click on) blank presentation. This would lead to another screen opening up, which would display various auto layouts. Select one of them, depending on the type of presentation to be made and click OK. The other options are using AutoContent Wizard or general template. For medical presentation these tools are less helpful.
5. For making any slide, you will need a background design, which is a beginner and easy to be selected from the standard design provided in the program. To select it, checkout the options given in the toolbar, on the top of the screen (there are various standard functions, one can use for making the presentation. If you keep the cursor on any option on the toolbar, a small title would appear and tell you about what function can be performed, when you click the mouse while keeping the cursor on it). A dark background with a white or light yellow font, or any other color with sharp contrasts enhances the legibility of the text slides.
6. Now, fill in the text on the slide by typing from your written text or you can copy and paste material from your notes prepared on the MS Word (or any other word program).
7. You can also select to change the font size and color of the text, clicking the cursor on the appropriate options on the toolbar, displayed at the top and bottom of the screen. The minimum desired font size for Times New Roman scripts is 28 points, for text and title the scripts is 40 points.

8. One can also select Arial or Verdana for the presentation, but avoid using different fonts in the same presentation. Fonts that are too thick (Verdana) or tend to merge with each other are best avoided. It is very important to be careful about spelling mistakes because they appear glaring when exhibited on a large screen.
9. Charts and tables can be created by choosing these options from the formatting toolbar. Insert table option with a preset number of rows and columns, while draw a table feature requires manual preparation of the tables.
10. The use or abuse of color can make or mark any presentation. Proper contrast between the color of background and text is of extreme importance for readability and impact of the slide. The slides can be embellished with headers, footers, charts, tables, graphs, etc. by making use of various options available on the formatting toolbar. If one needs to transfer some picture or graphic from other textual resource, then a scanner is required to generate its digital image. The scanned material can be pasted on the slide with appropriate placement.
11. Once a slide is ready, save it by clicking in the save option on the toolbar.
12. Once all the slides of the presentation have been created, one may wish to change the order of the slides, going in to slide sorter (in view menu) and can do this. The slide sorter would show all the slides in presentation, lined on the screen as thumbnails. Dragging a slide up or down to a desired location or number with the help of mouse can change the slide sequence to any particular order or cutting the slide and pasting it to the desired place can be done too.
13. Audio and video can also be added to the presentation.
14. The introduction of one slide after another can be done in various ways. This is called transition. The speed and style of transition needs to be checked and used in a consistent manner. A repeated and frequent change in the style of transition needs to be avoided. Over enthusiasm in this matter would lead to viewers being distracted.
15. The presentation, once ready, can be carried out to the venue on all laptop or compact disk (CD) or a Pen Drive. It is preferable to have the presentation on Pen Drive, which has larger memory space (so that you can keep all your presentations on it) and is

compatible to any machine as well. It may be good alternative to send the presentation through internet to an e-mail account, which can be accessed from anywhere and downloaded on the projecting computer.

USES OF DIGITAL IMAGE

Digital image is an extremely useful mode to enhance the presentation and improves the understanding of the subject to a large section of the audience. Pictures, graphs and illustrations should be carefully chosen to supplement the presentation. CD-ROM, digital cameras, mobile camera, scanners and internet are good sources, which can provide good graphics, but it is a good idea to check whether the image is protected by a copy right or not. It is also important to remember that graphics may occupy a large disk space and one should use the format (such as jpeg and gif) that takes less disk space. Also, if one uses figures, tables and graphs from the books and journals, the quality of these pictures gets downgraded in a step wise manner by photocopying. If one has to get good quality images, then a good quality camera or a scanner with a high resolution is desirable. Some tips for making effective PowerPoint presentation are shown in Box 8.1.

Box 8.1: Effective PowerPoint presentation

- Keep the information on slide simple and easy to follow
- Maintain consistency in color, text and background
- Use color to highlight and contrast
- Avoid over using special effects
- Handouts are helpful for audience to follow and take home messages
- Prepare and practice your presentation well, specially beeping in mind the time allotted

CONCLUSION

Creating a PowerPoint presentation is a reasonable easy proposition although in the beginning, it may appear to be difficult or confusing. Always remember that computer is a user-friendly machine and the more one works on it, the more savvy one would become in its use. Summarily a good PowerPoint presentation should have clarity, legibility and consistency as its top priority. A clear, consistent and focused MS PowerPoint presentation is a great asset to the speakers, who wants to put across his/her knowledge, thoughts and ideas to the target audience in the best possible way.

FURTHER READING

1. Available from http://presentations.com
2. Bradbury A. Successful Presentations Skills, 2nd edition. New Delhi: Kogan Page India; 2002. pp. 78-102.
3. Shendurnikar N, Goel Sanjeev. Medical presentations. In: Thacker Naveen (Ed). Computers for Doctors. New Delhi: Jaypee Brothers Medical Publishers (P) Ltd; 2003. pp. 105-15.

9

Understanding Mobile Operating Systems

Sanjeev Goel

INTRODUCTION

Mobile is no longer a status symbol. Gone are the days, when the mobiles were used only to make calls and occasionally used to send messages. Today's mobiles can perform almost all the functions of a computer such as sending e-mails, playing games, browsing internet, etc. All this is possible due to invention of smartphone, having an operating system (OS). The smartphones sell on basis of functionality of the mobile and it is their OS that defines what functions a mobile can carry out.

A mobile consists of just three blocks; the hardware, the operating system, and then all the software that runs on the OS. OS is the basic software of a mobile, which controls all its functions. It allows user to install and execute third party applications—popularly called apps. This helps to add new functionality to the mobile. Today's mobiles with proper OS are called smartphones. There is thousands of app available for download and constantly being developed with their own purpose. Users have wide choice of applications such as productivity apps, communication, entertainment, lifestyle, music, weather, games, digital maps, books, etc. Standardized OS platforms make it possible to provide a consistent user interface and experience across devices from different hardware manufacturers.

There is a little known fact that every mobile has two OS and the other small OS manages everything related to radio. This OS is stored in firmware, and runs on the baseband processor. The second OS is entirely proprietary and is not very well documented or reviewed and may not be safe, and that is why many people are not comfortable using mobile for financial transactions or for sensitive information.

WHAT DOES OPERATING SYSTEM DO?

Operating system is the brain of the smartphone. Different smartphones have different processors, different displays and different hardware. It is the OS, which will get the best out of them. It does so by deciding how much memory to be given to each app for running. It allows multiple apps to work simultaneously. Some OS called open source, allows the source code of the OS to be available to anyone who wants to develop app to install it on the mobile and add functionality to the mobile. One can no longer stuck with what the mobile manufacturer has provided.

TYPES OF OPERATING SYSTEMS

There are number of mobile OS available. Some are open source, while some are restricted. In open source, it has no restrictions on 'who develops it and who can download'. It is customizable. In restricted OS, there are restrictions between developers and the users. For example, open OS is Android, while iPhone OS (iOS), Symbian, BlackBerry are restricted OS. The mobile OS is determined by the manufacturer of the mobile and cannot be changed or replaced by the user.

Evolution of Mobile Operating System

The first OS was by Palm in 1996 and since then there is no looking back. Some companies developed their own OS with much fanfare, but had to discontinue them due to limited apps available for them, like Bada by Samsung. The fastest developing OS as on now is Android due to its open source and adaptation by many mobile manufacturing companies like Samsung, HTC, LG, etc. However, the maximum number of apps is still by iOS owned by Apple. The following table gives some insight into the development of evolution of OS. The Table 9.1 includes major OS and not all.

Although the history of OS dates back to 1996, it was only in the year 2007, when people took note of the OS. Till the first version of iPhone was introduced by Steve Jobs, nobody was really bothered as to what OS was on their mobile, so long as it did its job. It was big wows evoked by Steve Jobs creation that other companies took note and started developing their own OS and in 2008, Google developed its own OS Android. The others like BlackBerry, Samsung and Nokia also followed and started to improve their OS for providing better functionality to their mobiles.

Table 9.1: Evolution of operating systems

Year	Operating system	Comments
2003	Windows Mobile 2003	Bluetooth, Internet Explorer, Media Player 9
2004	Windows Mobile 2003	Landscape switching
	Palm OS Cobalt	Telecommunication, Bluetooth, Wi Fi
2005	Windows Mobile 5	Media Player 10, GPS*, MS† Office
	BlackBerry OS 4.1	
	Google acquired Android	
2007	First version of iPhone introduced	
	Windows Mobile 6	SQL‡-Server, Windows Live
	BlackBerry OS 4.5	Voice notes, e-mail, SMS§ in separate folders
2008	iOS 2.0	Third party-app support, Sync Google contacts
	BlackBerry OS 4.5	HTML‖, e-mails, faster and multitasking, MS‖ Office documents
	Windows Mobile 6.1	Threaded sms full page, zooming in
	Android 1.0	
	Symbian OS 1	Desktop app widgets, Facebook, IM¶ Chat
2009	Android 1.1	Saving attachments, API** Change
2009	BlackBerry OS 5	Wireless sync, revamped web browser
	Windows 6.5	Internet Explorer, Multi-Touch Support
	Samsung Bada 1.0	
	iOS 3.0	Push notification, cut, copy and paste, Voice Memos
	HP webOS	Multi touch gestures, multitasking
April 2009	Android 1.5 (Cupcake)	Bluetooth, uploading videos to YouTube

Contd...

Contd...

Year	Operating system	Comments
September 2009	Android 1.6 (Donut)	WVGA[††] screen resolution, Google free
Oct 2009	Android 2.0/2.1 (Éclair)	HTML 5 support, Bluetooth 2.1
2010	iOS 4.0	Multitasking, folders
	BlackBerry OS 6.0	New medic interphase, stronger social media, multiple contact lists and track pad support
	Android 2.2 (Froyo, Frozen Yogurt)	USB[‡‡] tethering, Wi-Fi hotspot, Adobe flash 10.1 support
	Windows 7	Tile UI[§§], cloud-based services and multitasking
	Android 2.3 (Gingerbread)	Multi-touch software keyboard, support for extra large screen sizes and resolutions
	Symbian 2	Royalty free version
	Symbian 3	Native WebKit-based browser, 2D and 3D graphics
2011	Android 3.0 (Honeycomb)	Optimized tablet support
2011	Android 4.0 (Ice Cream Sandwich)	New typeface called Robot, New face unlock feature, rearrange able folders, swipe to dismiss notifications, tasks and browser tabs, Wi-Fi Direct support
2012	Android 4.1 (Jelly Bean)	Faster, smoother more responsive, resizable apps widgets, offline voice dictation, better faster apps updates
2013	BlackBerry OS 10	Uses a combination of gestures and touches for navigation
	Android 4.4 (KitKat)	Better memory management to access app developers to target power and mobiles

*GPS, global positioning system; †MS, Microsoft; ‡SQL, structured query language, §SMS, short message service, ||HTML, hypertext markup language; ¶IM, instant message; **API, application programming interface; ††WVGA, wide video graphics array; ‡‡USB, universal serial bus; §§UI, user interface.

OPERATING SOFTWARE

There are many OS available in the market; the detailing of all of these are not within the scope of this chapter. We will be discussing iOS, Android, BlackBerry and Windows.

iPhone OS

The iPhone OS was introduced in the year 2007 by Apple Inc. initially used for mobile phone, now it is being used for iPhone, iPod Touch, iPad and generation TV. The initial versions were called iPhones and the first to be launched was OS X in 2010, Apple branded iPhone as iOS. The major updates are done almost once a year. The latest version is iOS 7.0, which is available for iPhone 4, iPhone 5, iPhone 5C, iPhone 5S and iPad 2. Initially third party applications were not allowed. It is the foundation of iPhone, iPad and iTouch. As it is not open source software, it does not allow iOS to set up on non-Apple products. As on date, there are more than 1 million apps available for iOS. The concept of iOS is direct contact with fingers, switches, buttons and gestures. The gestures include swipe, tap, pinch and reverse pinch. It can also work by shaking or rotating.

The home screen (rendered by and also known as 'SpringBoard') displays application icons and a dock at the bottom of the screen, where users can pin their most frequently used apps. The status bar is at the top. The rest of the screen is for current applications. In the latest versions, the icons of the apps can be placed on the home screen based on usability and appearance of home screen. There is a facility of creating folders, where a group of apps can be stored depending upon the users choice. The notifications for missed calls, messages, etc. are in the task bar and can be scrolled down. The bottom row of applications called dock contains are iPhone's main purposes. Originally phone, mail, Safari and iPod starting with iOS 5, the iPod app was split into two apps, music and videos, as it always has been on the iPod Touch, and the music app replaced the iPod app in the dock. In iOS 7, the iPhone gains a dedicated FaceTime app (previously integrated into the phone app), as it had been on the iPod Touch and iPad, since iOS 4. There is provision of multitasking and the apps can be updated automatically in the back ground. Siri is a voice-based intelligent personal assistant, which works as an application on supported devices. The service, directed by the user's spoken commands, can do a variety of different tasks, such as call or text someone, open an app, search the web, lookup sports information, find directions or locations, and answer general knowledge questions. There are game centers to play various games. In a major shift to allow third party apps, Apple gave software development kit (SDK) though which the apps could be developed. However to include the apps in the Apple store a developer program fee has to be given. The developer can distribute it free or sell it through Apple store. 70% of the fees go to the developer, while 30% is shared by Apple. There have been attempts by hackers to break (Jail breaking) into the system of iOS, but without much success. Most of the iOS platforms iPhones are locked and do not allow all the phones to be used by all the mobile operators. The iOS updates are free and one of the most secure OS.

Android Operating System

Android OS is based on Linux kernel and is primarily designed for touch screen smartphones. It was initially developed by Android and later taken over by Google in 2005. The first version of Android was released in the year 2008. The operation of the screen is mainly touch and is supported by swiping, pinching, reverse pinching, tilting, etc. It is open source OS and it can be freely modified, and distributed by device manufacturers, wireless carriers and developers. There are around 7 lacks apps available for android and it is said that it is the most preferred OS for the developers. It has overtaken Symbian and is likely to overtake iOS given its popularity and open source. It is already used on maximum number of smartphone platforms. As of November 2013, its share has increased to 80% of total market. In 2007 consortium of Google, mobile handset makers Sony, HTC and Samsung along with a few wireless carriers revealed launching of android. The first phone to use Android was HTC Dream released on October 22, 2008. The first version was Android 1.1. Subsequently there have been numerous updates. Each version is named after a dessert or a sugary treat. The versions are named in alphabetical order and the first one Android 1.5 was named Cupcake, followed by 1.6 Donut and now 4.4 KitKat, which was released in October 2013. It is as of now available in 46 languages.

Android requires minimum 512 MB of random access memory (RAM). Android devices are incorporating many optional hardware components, including still or video cameras, hardware orientation sensors, dedicated gaming controls, accelerometers, gyroscopes, barometers, magnetometers, proximity sensors, pressure sensors, thermometers and touch screens. The initial screen that opens on the mobile is home screen, which is like the desktop of a computer. The home screen contains apps icons and widgets. App icon on clicking opens the app, while the widget displays the live event such as weather, e-mails, news, clock, etc. the apps can be acquired from play store either free or by payment. Android has provision to automatically suspend the app, if it is not being used to save energy. This saves energy and the app can be restarted without wasting time. Android updates are available every 6-9 months.

Google provides free updates for up to 18 months of purchase of the mobile phone. The unlocked Android-based mobiles are available freely. Security is an issue with Android. Although the apps are stored separately in 'Sandbox' an isolated area of the mobile, most of the apps require the users to grant permission to use other functions of the mobile making it vulnerable to virus threats.

Although many antivirus software are available, they are not effective. The information on the mobile specially the address book can be accessed by malwares without the knowledge of the user. Android versions 4.2, Jelly Bean and above have inbuilt security in form of malware scanner. Android phone with the help of GPS can keep a tract of location of the mobile phone. There are security agencies, which have access to the data including SMS on the mobile.

Since, its launch in 2007, Android has grown to become the most widely used smartphone OS and 'one of the fastest mobile experiences available.' From a market share of 2.8% in 2008, it has grown to 80% in 2013 presented on Table 9.2.

Note that the names are all names of desserts and are arranged in alphabetical order.

Table 9.2: Versions of android

Name	Version	Released on
1.5	Cupcake	April 2009
1.6	Donut	September 2009
2	Eclair	October 2009
2.2	Froyo	May 2010
2.3.3–2.3.7	Ginger-bread	February 2011
3.1–3.2	Honey-comb	May 11
4.0.3–4.0.4	Ice cream Sandwich	December 2011
4.1–4.3	Jelly bean	July 12
4.4	KitKat	October 13

BlackBerry Operating System

BlackBerry OS is proprietary developed by Blackberry Ltd for its mobile phones. This OS can only be found on BlackBerry phones. It has unique system as OS is driven by track wheel, track ball, track pad and now recently touch screen. It is popular for its e-mail capabilities as the e-mails can be sync real time from its own dedicated BlackBerry Enterprise Server. The third party apps have to be digitally signed, making it one of the most secure OS. The updates are automatically available. The first BlackBerry OS version 1.0 was released in January 1999. The last version released is version 10.0, which has included a unique platform-wide flow interface, a new intelligent keyboard, as well as a camera app, which allows the user to time-adjust the whole photo and also time-adjust individual face, one at a time to optimize picture quality. It has also allowed FM radio on its OS. The latest version allows multitasking and gesture enabled navigation. It has camera, which takes multiple photos for the same subject, enabling the user to select the best possible picture. It also allows hotspot Wi-Fi. A unique feature of version 10 is that, it has allowed Android platform through which the user can download the third party apps for Android. The version for Android provided is 4.2 Jelly Bean. It supports sync, with computer via Wi-Fi. There are around 70,000 apps available for BlackBerry OS. As it has Android platform, all the apps of Android can also be downloaded. It has capabilities to work on MS Office files.

Windows Mobile Operating System

Window mobile is again a proprietary OS from Microsoft. The first version was launched in 2000. Windows mobiles are made by Nokia, HTC and some Samsung mobiles. The market share of Windows Mobile was 11% in 2004, which gradually rise to 42% in 2007. Then the decline started and at present, it has a market share of around 4%. The current version is 8, which was launched in October 2013. Most versions of Windows Mobile have a set of standard features, such as multitasking and the ability to navigate like in Windows OS of computers. It has most of the features available on other OS, but does not have call record, however a lot of information can be kept private, when using MS Office server instead of synchronization with other cloud servers.

CONCLUSION

As your decision of buying a mobile phone is based on the OS, it is important to know the OS, which your mobile phone has. If you have not bought the mobile phone, the manufacturer's specifications will tell you the OS and the version of the particular mobile phone. However, if you already have a mobile, the OS and the version can be found in the help or about menu in the settings of your mobile phone.

FURTHER READING

1. Available from http://www.android.com/
2. Available from http://en.wikipedia.org/wiki/BlackBerry 10
3. Available from http://en.wikipedia.org/wiki/Comparison_of_mobile_operating_systems
4. Available from http://en.wikipedia.org/wiki/Windows_Mobile

10

Smartphones and their Applications

Pritesh Nagar

INTRODUCTION

About a decade ago mobile phones were just a means of verbal communication between two persons and occasionally used for messaging. From then they have made progress in leaps and bounds and today the world is flooded with what we call 'smartphones'. There is no legal definition of a smartphone. It is a device which does communication in all forms, audio and video support, mail and internet support, calendars, documents, photographs, applications with a wide array of usefulness. The use of smartphone applications in health care is a boon, which can bring up to date information and patient care at bedside; at the point of care. Until now without these devices this kind of care delivery was not possible. It is imperative that healthcare professionals embrace this technological advancement and use it to improve quality of services to patients. Among the myriad of uses a smartphone can have for health care a few are:

1. Quick and ready access to healthcare information, references and medical tools, and calculators at point of care.
2. Improved nursing care with better accessibility to patient care tools and ready information.
3. Patient education and tools to monitor their disease conditions and lifestyle.
4. Though in nascent stages, smartphone-based bedside diagnostic devices such as ultrasound and electrocardiography (ECG) are not far from becoming a practicality.
5. Back-end management of electronic medical records and data management are also possible.

HISTORY

The first smartphone actually built was the IBM Simon in the year 1992. It was bulky and not fit for commercial use. The word 'Smartphone' was used by Ericsson in the year 1997. Just like a computer, a smartphone works on a mobile computing platform [operating system (OS)]. The earliest smartphones operated on the 'Palm' and the 'EPOC' OS. From 2000 till about 2007-2008, the 'Windows' and 'Symbian' OS dominated the smartphone Arena. From then Apple's 'iOS' and Google's 'Android' have completely dominated the smartphone ecosystem. Today more than three-quarters (75%) of the smartphones in the world are based on the Android platform by Google. Apple follows a distant second with about 20% share.

SMARTPHONE PENETRATION

According to the global smartphone application report 2010, more than 85% of doctors use a smartphone. However, only 30-50% doctors actually make use of smartphones in their clinical practice. However, this is very less information and statistics on the use of smartphones by nurses. In one US survey by Springer publishing company around 74.6% of the nurses owned a smartphone. About 43.7% owned an iPhone and 29.8% owned an Android device. However, nearly half of them had never used a medical application and all those who had used; were using only Epocrates. In the survey, 68% of the users never used or purchased an eBook. This shows that though there may be an increasing trend to use smartphones among all sections of population including health care, there is a lack of awareness or sparse usage of the same for point of care and healthcare delivery. There is a need to enhance the health care application of smartphones at all levels of personnel by providing education and technical assistance.

MEDICAL APPLICATIONS

Apple's iOS leads the pack of smartphone OS with maximum applications (close to 10,000) for health care personnel. Android comes in a distant second in the number (about 3,500) of health care related applications. However, when we compare most of the major and top most health care applications across the most of them are available on both the platforms. Most common and popularly used medical applications are given in Table 10.1.

Table 10.1: Commonly used medical applications

Application	Free	Android	iOS
Medscape	√	√	√
Prognosis	√	√	√
UpToDate	×	√	√
Micromedex	√	√	√
Visual body	×	×	√
Oxford clinical handbooks	×	√	√
Epocrates	√	√	√
Merck manual	×	√	√
Lexicomp	×	√	√
ECG* guide	×	√	√

*ECG, electrocardiography

Smartphone Applications for Nursing Care

The various apps of health care can be broadly classified into drug references, medical information references, medical calculators and lifestyle related apps. The latter are more useful for patients and general public, not healthcare professionals and may not be referenced form reliable sources all the time. The various apps useful for practice are grouped in separate categories and a brief discussion is mentioned in the following section.

All-in-one Applications

All-in-one application are an amalgamation of medical references, drug formulary and medical calculators. When opting for a general or a single application, these are the best bet to get all possible information in one place. Medscape, Skyscape and Lexicomp are the best known and reliable applications in this category.

Medscape brings to a smartphone, all the information that is available in the web version of the same. Most of the articles can be downloaded for offline reference, so that a working data connection is not required for the application to work. The built in drug reference is complete with both pediatric and adult dosing patterns, adverse effects, contraindications and drug interactions. There is also a built in medical calculator with formulae for most of the day-to-day needs of a clinician and nurse. It also brings latest medical news and gives the user to complete Medscape CMEs through the applications itself. It requires a working Medscape username and password to use the applications and it is completely free.

Epocrates is another application with features as good as Medscape. However it has free version and different grades of paid versions. To access all the features, the paid versions are needed which are available on an annual subscription basis. The free version does include drug references, medical calculators and a few medical references; albeit not as extensive Medscape.

Skyscape is another reliable provider of medical applications. The list of applications by Skyscape includes Skyscape Medical, Skyscape RxDrugs, Skyscape Primary Care Suite, Skyscape Dermatology and Skyscape Oncology. Among these Skyscape Medical is free and is the most downloaded, and used applications. The drug application is also free, but others need to be purchased and the prices are pretty steep. Skyscape Medical includes information on drugs, medical calculators and clinical information on quite a few topics. Here again the amount of information offered falls short of what Medscape has to offer. The application has built in feature to purchase more than 600 different medical resources spanning across 35 medical specialties. There is a Skyscape application on nursing procedures as well, but price is upwards rupees 4,000. Lexicomp has information mostly limited to drug references and related material.

Medical Calculators

Most of the above mentioned all-in-one applications offer medical calculators. However, there are some stand-alone medical calculators, which offer much more extensive information. 'Pediatric Oncall a very famous online site offers a free medical calculator, which includes the basic pediatric anthropometric calculations, as well as most of the needs of a pediatrician. For a more comprehensive calculator we need to look beyond. There are calculators available to address individual needs such as body mass index (BMI), intravenous (IV) drip rate calculator, pregnancy calculators, diabetes and renal problem related calculators.

The most extensive calculator is probably Mediquations. It has 232 medical formulae and scores with a facility for US and SI units. The formulae are grouped by categories and there is a facility to earmark most used scores and formulae. It is a paid application, but is not very expensive. MediCalc and Medical Calculator are two other applications, which are good, but they pale in comparison to number of options available in Mediquations.

Clinical Decision-making Tools

Unbound Medicine is one of the reputed mobile medical apps developers. It along with Skyscape has developed several applications by the name of '5-Minute Consult'. These applications are spread over a wide variety of fields such as medicine, pediatrics, emergency medicine, orthopedics and neurology. They are a quick reference for making a diagnosis in a very rapid access format. Based on the diagnosis, there are standard recommendations for investigations and therapeutic regimens. The information is laid out in tables and algorithms, and is easy to follow. The downside is that all of these applications are very steeply priced.

Diagnosaurus is another application in this category. It would not be a true clinical decision-making tool, because there are no algorithms here. It is very basic and gives a differential diagnosis for a particular symptom. Beyond that it offers nothing.

The Merck Manual is another excellent application. It could be called crossover between a medical reference apps and clinical decision-making tool. Again the subscription prices are very high.

Dictionaries

Taber's and Dorland's dictionary are probably the best ones out there, but both of them require purchase. Both of them are almost equal in content and ease of use, but Dorland's is half the price of Taber's. Merriam-Webster is an alternative free medical dictionary.

Specific Nursing Applications

Mosby's Nursing Consult is published by Elsevier, a reputed medical publisher. It is a paid application and requires institutional subscription. It offers a very good combination of drug monographs, drug calculators, evidenced-based nursing monographs and patient education material.

Nursing Essentials is another paid apps, but the price is very less and affordable. It is a very comprehensive apps providing vital information related to almost all specialties and across all age groups. It provides updated reference information on drugs, infusions and laboratory values, with information on medications, blood products, calculations and per OS (PO), subcutaneous (SC), intramuscular (IM), intraosseous (IO) administration procedures, with a section on IV administration guidelines. It also features information on fluids, electrolytes, acid-base imbalances, pain assessment chart, pediatric and geriatric considerations, burns and dermatome charts, neurological and psychiatric assessments, immunizations, medical procedure and a host of other things. It is probably one of the most values for money exclusive nursing apps that one can purchase.

Nursing Drug Handbook by Lippincott is complete nursing information on drugs and related matters. The drawback is that only 25 monograms are available in the free version and rest need to be purchased from within the applications.

Nurse's Drug Handbook TR is from McGraw-Hill and is another paid drug application meant for nurses. Notable features in this application apart from routine are a 32 page insert on safe drug administration and critical advice related to treatment of adverse drug reactions.

Nursing Diagnosis Handbook is from Unbound Medicine and is another excellent apps, albeit paid and steeply priced. It primarily contains essential information required to reach an accurate nursing diagnosis and formulate nursing care plans. The user has access to about 1,300 signs and symptoms, medical diagnosis and surgical matters. From this information there is link and information provided to detailed nursing care plans. Information and reference links to PubMed database make the application even more useful.

CONCLUSION

Smartphones will continue to play a very important role in our medical lives. They are not only useful for clinicians but also for nurses, paramedical staff and patients. However, it is very important to choose a medical app, which is from a reliable source and a reputed publisher; it is free of conflicts of interest and with proper reference resource. When using patient data with medical applications; importance to patient information confidentiality should be given and adhered to. Use of applications with a critical appraisal of their benefits and harms in a balanced manner will help us all a lot in delivering better, up-to-date and technically sound service to our patients.

FURTHER READING

1. Edwards J, O'Connor PA. Improving technological competency in nursing students: The passport project. The Journal of Educators Online. 2011;8(2):1-20.
2. Mosa As, Yoo I Sheets L. A systematic review of healthcare applications for smartphones. BMC Med Inform and Decis Mak. 2012;12:67.
3. Odiodu V, Odiodu E. An empirical review of the top 500 medical apps in a European Android market. Journal MTM. 2012;1(4):22-37.
4. Visser BJ, Bouman J. There's a medical app for that. Student BMJ. 2012;20:e2162.
5. White A, Allen P, Goodwin L, et al. Infusing PDA technology into nursing education. Nurse Educ. 2005;30(4):150-4.
6. Wyatt T, Krauskopf P. E-health and Nursing: Using Smartphones to Enhance Nursing Practice. OJNI 2012;16(2).

11

Internet Search for Medical Literature and Resources

Niranjan Shendurnikar, Paresh Thakkar

INTRODUCTION

In this era of internet the world has become a global village. The necessary information can be availed easily by searching on internet and also is true in searching for medical literature. While doing, so it is often difficult to decide for the most appropriate and useful information out of huge load of information available through internet. This problem can overcome by learning how to do 'effective search' for medical literature on internet. This is an era of 'evidence-based medicine (EBM)' and aim of search is to find the evidence. The term evidence-based medicine first appeared in year 1990 and today all healthcare providers have to practice based on the best evidence currently available called evidence-based health care or evidence-based practice. It has caused substantial shifted medical paradigm from traditional unsystematic clinical experience to findings of evidence-based research.

HIERARCHY OF EVIDENCE

While doing the literature search, one should be aware about the nature and strength of the evidence and the hierarchy of evidence (Box 11.1).

Box 11.1: Hierarchy of strength of evidence for treatment decisions

- Systematic reviews of randomized trials
- Single randomized trial
- Systematic review of observational studies addressing patient important outcomes
- Single observational study addressing patient important outcomes
- Physiologic studies of (blood pressure, cardiac output, exercise capacity bone density and so forth)
- Unsystematic clinical observations

The findings of unsystematic clinical observations may suffer from bias, which can be minimum in randomized control trials. While a single randomized controlled trial (RCT) may still suffer from bias or methodological flaws, systematic reviews of multiple RCT can guard against such misleading results. There are certain preprocess information available, which have been reviewed and critically analyzed. The following is the hierarchy of the preprocessed evidence (Box 11.2).

Box 11.2: Hierarchy of preprocessed evidence

1. **Studies:** Preprocessing involves selecting only those studies that are both highly relevant and characterized by study designs that minimize bias and thus permit a high strength of inference.
2. **Systematic reviews:** It provide clinicians with an overview of all of the evidence addressing a focused clinical question.
3. **Synopses:** Of individual studies or of systematic reviews encapsulated the key methodological details and results required to apply the evidence to individual patient care.
4. **Systems:** Practice guidelines, clinical pathways or evidence-based textbook summaries of a clinical area provide the clinicians with much of the information needed to guide the care of individual patients.

Finding the Evidence

A paramedical student or medical student early in their training hardly consults the original medical literature. In the early part of training their focus is to learn and understand normal human physiology, pathophysiology associated with patients' condition or problem. After having grasped these basic concepts, they are faced with problem solving of patient-related problems in day-to-day practice. Such problem solving questions are more precise and address specific issues in management of patients. So, this demands skill of formulating appropriate questions.

Browsing vs Problem Solving

Surfing the internet for a target, medical journals relevant to one's specialty, which can be called browsing mode has a major limitation of inefficiency and might end up in frustration. The questions raised in management of patients' are defined and the literature search is done to solve the problem. This will give more precise information from the overwhelming amount of literature available.

Browsing

Browsing for medical literature may not yield the precise information for patients' management, but often required for primary information for new topics or for getting an overall idea about the medical topic. Less than 10% of articles published in core medical journals are of both high quality and of clinically utility. One efficient strategy can be restricting browsing to secondary journals for example, internal and general medicine, American College of Physician (ACP) journal club, which publishes synopsis of articles, which are both clinically relevant and methodologically sound. While doing the web browsing, one must evaluate the authenticity of the information available at a particular website.

Look at websites that provide reviews of health and medical internet resources such as network mapper and HealthWeb. It is a good idea to examine the resources in detail, looking at the home page, parent documents about the pages, help files, frequently asked questions (FAQ) and aims. Many groups interested in health and medical information on the internet produce evaluation guidelines that one can view online and use to help assess the quality of internet medical information. The examples of these include:

1. Biomedical (BioMed) evaluation guidelines.
2. British medical journal review.
3. Health on the net code of conduct: These are eight stringent criteria, mainly based on the health on the net (HON) code of conduct for health and medical websites and are used to evaluate medical information on the internet. A site with HON code certification will have the emblem of HON code on its homepage and can be considered authentic. The site could also be considered safe for using the credit card for online payments.

Use of Search Engines

Search engines are websites that allow to search the internet or specific parts of it by typing in a topic.

Medical Search Engines

1. **MD's choice:** A good search engine looking for medical topics on the internet (search—acute otitis media).

2. **MedHunt:** Health on the Net Foundation medical web search engine (will indicate number of sites with HON code certification).
3. **Medical World Search:** Another search engine for looking for medical topics on the internet. This requires subscription. Others are Health on the Net, Medical Matrix, MedWebPlus, Vivisimo, BioMed and Yahoo Health.

Metasearch Engines

These search engines will take the subject and search several other search engines to find web pages. They will often find more sites than a general search engine, such as:

1. **Google:** It ranks the results of by popularity.
2. **Carnic.com:** Logo of this site is 'what you need, when you need it?
3. **Yahoo:** Gives excellent results and images.

QUICK REFERENCES TO DISEASES

MD Consult

MD consult provides evidence-based information related to diseases and has links to journals and books. The information related to diseases are divided into summary, background, diagnosis, treatment, outcome, prevention and resources. Other quick reference sites are DynaMed, eMedicine and InfoRetriever. Following are few of the sites of interest for nurses, midwives and health visitors.

Internet Orientation: Good to Start

The following are good to start internet resources for nursing health professionals:

1. **Nursing, Midwifery and Allied Professions (NMAP):** It is a good place to start. This is a United Kingdom (UK) based subject gateway to quality nursing, midwifery and allied health information on the internet. All sites found through this gateway have been evaluated and indexed and come with a brief description that enables to assess their usefulness before the visit.
2. **National Electronic Library for Health (NeLH):** Provides access to a range of resources. It also includes branch libraries for various conditions and professional portals for different

professional groups including nursing, midwifery and community practitioners.

Fact Finding on the Internet

For finding factual information about a disease, procedure or drugs the following web sources are of help:

1. **MedlinePlus:** Fore drug information, this is free site and provides information on generic drugs, products, side effects, dosage and treatment possibilities. It is also fully searchable.
2. **Searchable online version:** This is a free searchable online version of the widely used book. Published jointly by the British Medical Association and the Royal Pharmaceutical Society of Great Britain, aims to provide healthcare professionals with information about the use of medicines.
3. **Indian Academy of Pediatrics (IAP) drug formulary:** This is IAP recommendations for pediatric illnesses and monographs of drugs used in pediatrics are available as a book and searchable compact disk-read only memory (CD-ROM). Details of how to get a copy is available on the website.
4. **National Institute for Health and Care Excellence (NICE):** The NICE provides national guidance and advice to improve health and social care (www.nice.org.uk). The institute provides independent and evidence-based clinical guidelines on management of individual conditions, technology appraisals of cost-effectiveness of health technologies, social care guidance, which provides practical support to practitioners working with children and adult's social services and public health guidance. They also provide access to range of information, includes NICE evidence and online search engine that identifies relevant clinical, social care and public heath guidance. It also provides access to range of bibliographic databases such as MEDLINE and professional journals. It provides access to British National Formulary (BNF) and British National Formulary for Children (BNFC).

ONLINE LITERATURE SEARCH

If one is interested in a particular subject (for an essay, research project) and looking for articles that have been written in the past 5,

10 or 20 years search a bibliographic database for details of relevant articles before tracking down the journals and articles are in the internet has the capabilities to be used for both these tasks.

Bibliographic Databases for Nursing Professionals

Bibliographic databases are available with subscription only, but the free access may be if the Institution's Library subscribes to these sites:

1. **Cumulative Index of Nursing and Allied Health Literature (CINAHL):** Indexes the nursing and allied health literature from 1982 to the present, including over 1,500 nursing and allied health journals. Abstracts are included for some journal titles.
2. **British Nursing Index (BNI):** This index, produced by a network of libraries, covers mainly articles in English language from over 220 nursing and allied health journals (with an emphasis on British publications). The full service is available on the internet and CD-ROM by subscription only.
3. **Midwives Information and Resource Service (MIDIRS):** This gathers information from over 550 international journals and commissions original articles on the hot topics being discussed by the midwifery professionals. Subscribers to the MIDIRS, Midwifery Digest have access to the MIDIRS bibliographic database and around 400 preprepared standard subject searches.

Once bibliographic references are received from MEDLINE, CINAHL or BNI you will then want to track down the full-text articles from online electronic journals such as Journal of Community Nursing, which provides the full text of all articles and a search facility, but most electronic journals charge a subscription fee and require a password in order to gain full-text access.

Operating in Problem-solving Mode

The questions raised in management of patients are defined and the literature search is done to solve the problem. This will give more precise information from the overwhelming amount of literature available.

Framing the Question

Dissecting the questions into the component parts to find the best evidence is fundamental EBM skill. Most of the questions can be divided into following three parts:

1. Population means, who are relevant patients?
2. Exposure or interventions, one may be interested in knowing harmful effect of particular exposure leading to a particular condition such as smoking and lung cancer. One might be interested in effect or side effect of a particular intervention.
3. Outcome.

Initial question: Fluid management in patients of severe acute malnutrition coming with diarrhea.

Improved question (searchable question): These would specify relevant patient population, management strategy and consequence:

1. Patients, children with severe acute malnutrition with diarrhea.
2. Intervention of fluid therapy.
3. Outcomes are morbidity and mortality.

Framing a good searchable question would require an in-depth understanding of the clinical issues involved in the patient management and a careful thought, what one really wants to know. Once the question is framed, the next step is to translate the question into an effective search strategy.

Searching for the answer: For this one first needs to determine the type of question. Fundamentally there are four types of questions. Questions pertaining to:

- Therapy
- Harm
- Diagnosis
- Prognosis.

For this one also should have basic knowledge of types of studies, such as randomized control trial, observational studies, etc.

Sources of Evidence

Online resources are easier to search compared to print products. Table 11.1 gives online medical information resource contact information; few of them are paid.

Table 11.1: Medical information resources

Resources	Internet address
Cochrane Library	www.cochrane.org
UpToDate	www.uptodate.com
MEDLINE	www.medline.com
PubMed	www.pubmed.gov
Other sources	
Best evidence	www.medmatric.org www.acponline.org
Emedicine	www.emedicine.com
Medscape	www.medscape.com
Clinical practice guidelines	www.guidelines.gov
MD consult	www.mdconsult.com
Evidence-based medicine reviews (Ovid)	www.ovid.com
American College of Physician (ACP) Journal club	www.acpjc.org

Selection of the Best Medical Information Resource

Medical information will mainly depend upon the type of question, time available and access to the resources. Questions related to therapy, harm, diagnosis and treatment one can search through the databases such as MEDLINE, Best Evidence and UpToDate, while Cochrane Library can provide answers for questions pertaining to therapy RCT, meta-analysis and systematic reviews).

Using Prefiltered Medical Information Sources

Prefiltered means someone has reviewed the literature and chosen only the methodologically strongest studies and have designed them in such a way so as to make searching easy. The sources are updated regularly. Such sources are Cochrane library, UpToDate and Clinical Evidence.

Best Evidence

The best evidence provides quickest route to systematic reviews and original studies that address to focused clinical questions. It is a cumulative electronic version of ACP Journal Club and EBM. It is paid resource. This provides structured abstracts of studies that meet quality criteria along with accompanying commentary by an expert.

Cochrane library: The Cochrane Collaboration is an international organization that prepares, maintains and provides systematic reviews of healthcare interventions. They focus primarily on systematic reviews of controlled trials of therapeutic interventions. To search the Cochrane library, after logging onto the website, click on 'search' and then enter appropriate terms, which should be searched. Using the advance search option, you can create more complex search strategy that include medical subject headings (MeSH) and logical operators, which will narrow down search and give the more precise results.

UpToDate: Is an online textbook, which is well-referenced. It gets updated every 4 months.

Unfiltered Medical Information Sources

MEDLINE is a wonderful bibliographic database by National Library of Medicine (NLM). It has comprehensive coverage of medical journals and is readily accessible free of charge using PubMed. The United State (US) NLM provides a free access to a searchable database; more than 23 millions citations for biomedical literature from MEDLINE, life science journals and online books. The citations may include links to full text content from PubMed central and publisher websites. MeSH is the NLM controlled vocabulary thesauruses used for indexing the articles for PubMed. Largely, only abstracts and citations are available, but length full articles/links to these are also available.

Searching PubMed effectively will require knowledge of how the database is structured and how publications are indexed. One must know how to use MeSH, which will be text word searching and the use of logical operators such as AND and OR to combine different search results. For learning this, one may go to the PubMed website and learn through the tutorials.

Other Online Sources for Nursing Professionals

Electronic Books

Electronic books (E-books) have several advantages over print books:

- Provide 24 hour off-campus access
- Cannot be overdue; hence, no fines
- No limit on how many e-books one can access at once
- Provide value-added functionality such as keyword searching.

However, most of these books either need a subscription or a network user name and a password to access these resources. Some examples of medical textbooks available on the web are:

1. **Merck Manual of Diagnosis and Therapy:** This is a key example of a printed book in electronic form. Full text and tables are accessible, the whole publication is searchable by keyword and it is free.
2. **Electronic Textbook of Dermatology:** This is a virtual textbook that has full text including images throughout its chapters and is also free.
3. **Medicalstudent.com:** This is a digital library of authoritative medical information for all students of medicine.

Health News

The internet is a great place to find uptodate health news, which gets updated daily or weekly.

Online News Services

1. Centers for Disease Control (CDC) and Prevention focuses on developing and applying disease prevention and control, environmental health, health promotion and education activities designed to improve the health.
2. British Broadcasting Corporation (BBC) news health has a collection of articles on various health topics.
3. Nursing standard includes online items of news and analysis from the journal.
4. The site of the World Health Organization (WHO) gives information on its strategies to combat a plethora of health issues.
5. Scanning through the United Nations International Children's Emergency Fund (UNICEF), site also keeps health professionals updated on various health issues and disease outbreaks of children the world over.

Organizations

Most organizations have a space on their website for news and current developments where one can pick up some useful information such as child health and diseases, growth monitoring, nutrition, vaccinations and parenting issues. The example of such organizations include WHO, UNICEF, American Academy of Pediatrics (AAP), American Academy of Family Physicians (AAFP), National Polio Surveillance Project (NPSP), Mayo Clinic and many more.

Teaching and Learning Materials

There are many web resources that support health and medical teaching and learning.

Learning Materials

1. Head start in biology free internet course aimed at nursing students unfamiliar with biology. One must register, but access is free.
2. Electrocardiography (ECG) simulator generates 26 of the most common cardiac rhythms, which can be started and stopped by the user. There is also a game to test the knowledge. The site requires the Flash 4.0 'plug in' and can run over the internet or downloaded in Windows personal computer (PC) or media access control (Mac) formats. It is provided by SkillStat, a commercial company providing learning tools for nurses and paramedics.

Teaching Materials

Many organizations and individuals now provide PowerPoint presentations, which can be downloaded, some even give permission for them to be used or adapted for teaching, but there are a range of other resources, which could be useful:

1. **Bristol Biomedical Image Library:** This is a collection of over 8,500 veterinary, dental and medical images. This site aims to provide lecturers, teachers and researchers with access to downloadable images that they can use in lectures and seminars.

2. **Essentials of Human Anatomy and Physiology:** Designed to accompany the book 'Essentials of Human Anatomy and Physiology', which includes quizzes, case studies, weblinks and resources for instructors including lecture outlines and transparencies.
3. **Check out Amedeo (www.amedeo.com):** Have all the latest articles and their abstracts e-mailed every month on any topics of choice.

CONCLUSION

As this is an era of information technology, one has to master how to best utilize the information by learning how to do 'effective search of medical literature'. This can be acquired by knowledge of the resources and skills to get maximum benefit from these resources. This will not only save valuable time of healthcare providers but also enable them to practice evidence-based health care.

FURTHER READING

1. An Introduction. CI Stems School of Computing. New Delhi: Tata McGraw-Hill Publishing Company Ltd. 1999. pp 24-33.
2. Unni Jeeson. The wonderful world of Pubmed. CPU Bull CMEGIAP: March; 2004.
3. Gordon Guyatt, Drummond Rennie. Users' Guide to the Medical Literature-essentials of Evidence Based Clinical Practise. USA: JAMA and Archives Journals; 2004.

12

Multimedia

Maansi Ramnani, Upant Rao Dongre

DEFINING MULTIMEDIA

Multimedia is the creation of content which combines different elements such as image, text, audio, video, graphics and animation.

- It is a means of communication using multiple forms of elements to present information.
- It is used in computer to present information or content which constitute a mix of text, audio, graphics, animations and videos in a single content.

TYPES OF MULTIMEDIA

- **Text:** Type of information synthesized by computers which is appropriate for the target audience and easy to read, involving newspapers, magazines, headlines from news channels, etc.
- **Audio:** Sound, music, speech, etc.
- **Image:** Photo or pictures
- **Video:** Moving images: movie
- **Graphics and Animation:** Include cartoonish images to convey messages easily and quickly.

USES OF MULTIMEDIA

- Multiple media is used to enrich our communication or presentation
- The application of multimedia can be found in various spheres of life including but not limited to communication, e-learning and online learning courses, digital libraries, virtual training, telemedicine.
  - **Communication:** Multimedia offers powerful means of communication. It shows what things look like, how they move and how they change keeping an audience's interest,

establishing personal contact establishing the identity and academic credibility of a speaker and communicating the speaker's enthusiasm for the subject.

- **E-learning and online learning courses:** E-learning is learning conducted via electronic media, typically on the Internet. It includes recorded or broadcast lectures, demonstrating nursing procedures and techniques that learners will have to try themselves later, recording students' performances to enable feedback and promote reflection.
- **Digital libraries:**
  - A digital library is a special library with a focused collection of digital objects that can include text, visual and audio material, stored as electronic media formats along with means for organizing, storing, and retrieving the files and media contained in the library collection.
  - Digital libraries can vary immensely in size and scope. It can be maintained by individuals and organizations. It can be affiliated with established physical library buildings or academic institutions.
  - An electronic library is a type of information retrieval system. The digital content may be stored locally, or accessed remotely via computer networks.
- **Virtual training:** Nurses can get trained by looking at a virtual nursing procedures before practicing the same in real life conditions. It also helps the nurses to develop techniques and improve skills to enhance nursing care.
- **Telemedicine:** Telemedicine is much more than just teleconferencing. Many telemedicine applications are used with guaranteed quality of service.

FURTHER READING

1. Wikipedia, https://en.wikipedia.org/wiki/Multimedia
2. www.young-train.net
3. ACM Digital Library, dl.acm.org

13

Social Networking

Jeeson Unni, Sachidanand Kamath

INTRODUCTION

As the use of information and communication technology, and the internet continues to grow in all regions of the world, online social networks have emerged as the new way in which people connect socially. These services make it possible to interact via the web with those who share common interests and activities across political, economic, and geographic borders, keep in touch with family and friends and at times reach out to long lost friends. Various organizations of the user's profession may also be contacted for clarifying doubts and management issues. The leader among these sites as of today is Facebook with over 1.4 billion members. Data generated by recent surveys on usage of social networking sites, which highlights the fact that 58% of the world's population is accessing these sites is detailed in Table 13.1.

DEFINITION

Social media is defined as 'a group of internet-based applications that build on the ideological and technological foundations, and that allow the creation and exchange of user-generated content'. Social media may be categorized into six main types:

1. Collaborative projects (e.g. Wikipedia).
2. Blogs and microblogs (e.g. Twitter).
3. Content communities (e.g. YouTube).
4. Social networking sites (e.g. Facebook).
5. Virtual game worlds (e.g. World of Warcraft) and virtual social worlds (e.g. Second Life).

SOCIAL MEDIA AND PUBLIC HEALTH COMMUNICATION

The World Health Organization (WHO) has a Facebook page, a Twitter feed and a significant presence on YouTube. WHO is using

Table 13.1: Social networking statistics

Social networks	Percent (if yes)
Do you ever use/have a profile on (poll taken in early 2012) the following?	
Any social network	58%
Facebook	56%
LinkedIn	14%
Twitter	11%
Google+	9%
Social network statistics	**Data**
Total number of Facebook users worldwide	1.4 billion
Total percentage of 18–24 years old who already use social media	98%
Total percentage of people on earth who use Facebook	11%
Total amount of minutes people spend on Facebook every month	700 billion
Average amount of time a person uses Facebook per month	15 hour 33 minute
Total amount of people who access Facebook with phone	250 million
Total amount of websites that have integrated with Facebook	2.5 million
Total pieces of content shared on Facebook each month	70 billion
Total amount of unique YouTube users per month	490 million
Total amount of YouTube page views per month	92 billion
Total amount hours spent on YouTube per month	2.9 billion
Total amount of articles hosted by Wikipedia	17 million
Total number of active registered Twitter users	554,750,000
Number of new Twitter users signing up every day	135,000
Number of unique Twitter site visitors every month	190 million
Average number of tweets per day	58 million
Number of Twitter search engine queries everyday	2.1 billion
Percent of Twitter users who use their phone to tweet	43%
Number of active Twitter users every month	115 million

networking sites to disseminate public health information, to counter rumors and to keep public informed during disease outbreaks or disasters.

USE OF SOCIAL NETWORKING SITES IN NURSING

Networking with peers is essential to professional growth and career success. Social networking sites are making it easier for nurses around the world to share professional advice/experiences, ask questions, and stay informed about new job opportunities and advancements in their field. There are now around 355,000 registered nurses and midwives on Facebook in the UK alone. Some sites for nurses are given below.

Nurse Company

With a clean, classic interface, the nurse company.com is essentially Facebook for nurses. It comes with many of the social networking tools that Facebook provides, like a profile, wall and even friend suggestions for nurses you might know. Similar to Facebook, can post photos, start groups and comment on friends' statuses. This is a perfect way to increase the size of the professional network, while keeping it organized, and on a platform that is accessible and familiar.

Nurse Together

The articles, blogs, forums and job listings found on Nurse Together.com all speak to the sentiment that the website's name suggests nursing is a community effort. Nurse Together is an excellent place for nurses to seek out both professional and lifestyle advice. In the 'education' section, nursing students can find useful tips about the process of becoming a nurse, as well as information on the many career different paths, a nursing degree opens up.

Ultimate Nurse

The forum on UltimateNurse.com is an excellent place for novice and veteran nurses to find information about technical developments in the field, job openings and nursing news. By creating a username and password, one can log into Ultimate Nurse to read and comment on the thousands of threads covering topics such as licensed practical nurse (LPN) vs registered nurses (RN) vs Bachelor of Science in Nursing (BScN) and nursing education news.

Facebook and Twitter

Although not catered specifically to nurses, the social network Behemoths Facebook and Twitter offer great resources for nurses looking to connect with their colleagues. Facebook group pages like Nurse Rounds and Nursing life, and Twitter feeds like @NurseZone and @RNCentral all provide a place online for nurses to learn online, interact or even just vent. Twitter chats like #RNchat and #hcsm designate a specific time and date in which healthcare professionals come together to talk about issues that matter to them. Through Facebook and Twitter, one can even start their own online nursing community—one that may eventually come to help the fellow nurses as much as the aforementioned sites can help.

All India Nursing Association

Facebook page of the Indian association (https://www.facebook.com/aaina.india.in?ref=stream) was founded recently. All nursing students, nurses, midwives in India need to become its member, so that they can chat, discuss and post the views regarding nursing.

POLICY AND GUIDANCE DOCUMENTS RELATED TO SOCIAL MEDIA FOR NURSES

Since these sites provide increased opportunities to communicate at personal and professional levels, and an enhanced access to information by both healthcare providers and members of the public, some caution is required in the way a person 'behaves' on these sites. Professional, ethical, regulatory and legal issues need to be addressed. For nursing, this is evidenced by the growing volume of policy and guidance documents that focus on the use of social media. Some examples are given in Table 13.2.

Risks of Social Networking Sites

The worldwide concerns regarding uninhibited use of these sites include unmoderated content, privacy violation, unprofessional behavior and organizational risk.

Table 13.2: Examples of policy and guidance documents related to social media for nurses

Organization	Resources
American Nurses Association (ANA)	Social Networking Principles Toolkit (ANA, 2011) includes a statement of principles, a webinar, a fact sheet, a tip card, and a tips section about the use of social media (www.nursingworld.org/socialnetworkingtoolkit.aspx)
National Council of State Boards of Nursing (NCSBN)	White Paper: A Nurses Guide to the Use of Social Media (NCSBN, 2011) and other documents related to social media are available on the following website https://www.ncsbn.org/2930.htm
Nursing and Midwifery Council (NMC)	Advice Sheet on Social Networking (NMC, 2011). Available from www.nmc-uk.org/Nurses-and-midwives/Advice-by-topic/A/Advice/Social-networking-sites/

The inability to decipher what is genuine information from the unmoderated distribution of information on these sites may lead to bad decisions by both healthcare providers and members of the public.

There have been cases of nurses violating privacy of patients by putting confidential information of their patients on social networking sites and being punished for the same.

In addition to breaches of privacy and unprofessional behavior one needs to avoid include bullying of colleagues (or for students, bullying of other students); online criticism of colleagues or employers; and unprofessional behavior that may be in breach of codes of conduct. One could get sued for such conduct online. Employers run the risk of loss of reputation by inappropriate online behavior.

Practical Guidance for Students, Nurses and Midwives Using Social Networking Sites

The standard conduct, both online and offline, is important. These are follows:

1. Identify yourself as a nurse or midwife on Facebook and act responsibly at all times to uphold the reputation of the profession.

2. Do not use social networks to build or pursue relationships with patients and service users, even if they are no longer in your care. On receipt of a friendship request from a current or former patient, Facebook allows you to ignore the request without the person being informed, thus avoiding unnecessary embarrassment.
3. Do not discuss work-related issues online, including conversations about patients or complaints about colleagues. Even when anonymously posted, they are likely to be inappropriate.
4. Never post pictures of patients or service users, even if they ask you to do this. If your mobile phone has a camera, you should not use it in the workplace.
5. Social networking sites should not be used for raising and escalating concerns (commonly referred to as whistle blowing).
6. Protect your own privacy. Decide what information about yourself you want share and with whom, and adjust your privacy settings. On Facebook, you can adjust your privacy settings at group level to share different levels of information with different kinds of friends. Remember that the more your personal life is exposed through social networking sites, the more likely it is that this could have a negative impact.
7. Remember that everything you post online is public, even with the strictest privacy settings. Once something is online, it can be copied and redistributed, and it is easy to lose control of it. Presume that everything you post online will be permanent and will be shared.
8. You can take action if you find yourself the target of complaints or abuse on social networking sites. You can remove someone from your friend list and block them from interacting with you, and most sites will include mechanisms to report abusive activity and provide support for users who are subject to abuse by others.
9. If you are very concerned about someone else's behavior online, you should take steps to raise your concern, including if necessary with their university or employer. In the most serious circumstances, for example, if someone's use of a social networking site is unlawful, you should also report the incident to the police.

Additional Guidance for Employers and Educators

Do not advocate blanket bans on nurses, midwives or students joining, or using social networking sites as they are both unenforceable and counterproductive. Support the responsible use of social networking sites by them.

Healthcare providers and universities can derive benefits from these sites as their corporate presence they would lend credibility when engaging students, nurses and midwives dealing with various issues. Organizations should set out clear policies for staff and students on their use of social networking sites, encouraging responsible use.

Organizations should ensure those managers and those responsible for enforcing policies on social networking sites, understand them and apply them consistently, particularly if they are handling complaints.

Complaints about the use of social networking sites or other online activity should be taken as seriously as real-world events. Cyber-bullying for example, can be intrusive and distressing, and sharing confidential information online can be more damaging than sharing it verbally. When considering the circumstances of a complaint involving online activity, it can be useful to make a direct comparison with a real-world activity to ensure the seriousness of the complaint is judged appropriately.

CONCLUSION

Social networking is the in thing today and nurses need to be familiar with the reliable sites for nursing professionals, its advantages, cautions for working on them and thereby gain maximum utility from these facilities.

FURTHER READING

1. Barry J, Hardiker N. Advancing nursing practice through social media: a global perspective. Online J Issues Nurs. 2012;17(3):5.
2. Canadian Nurse Protective Society. Social media. Info LAW. 2010;19(3).
3. Cronquist R, Spector N. Nurses and social media: Regulatory concerns and guidelines. Journal of Nursing Regulation. 2011;2(3):37-40.
4. Jones B. Mixed uptake of social media among public health specialists. Bull World Health Organ. 2011;89:784-5.

5. Kaplan AM, Haenlein M. Users of the world, unite! The challenges and opportunities of Social Media. Business Horizons. 2010;53: 59-68.
6. Social Networking Statistics. [online]. Available from http://www.statisticbrain.com/social-networking-statistics/[Accessed on September 2013].
7. Twitter Statistics. [online]. Available from http://www.statisticbrain.com/twitter-statistics/ [Accessed on September 2013].

14

Patient Education and Information Technology

Mukesh Kumar Singh, Niranjan Shendurnikar

INTRODUCTION

Advances in information technology (IT) have introduced new design approaches that support healthcare delivery and patient education. Such advances enable a fundamental redesign of healthcare processes based on the use and integration of electronic communication at all levels. Healthcare IT has the potential to empower patients and support a transition from a role in which the patient is the passive recipient of care services to an active role in which the patient is informed and has choices, and involved in the decision-making process.

The world of healthcare is developing rapidly, carrying in its wake an obligation to provide the highest standards of care. Patients enjoy a better quality of life and recover more effectively, when they are knowledgeable about their care protocols. Understanding on the part of the patient enhances adherence to prescribed treatment and this is particularly true of the common chronic diseases such as asthma, epilepsy, migraine, diabetes and hypertension. Patients also need 'information' to make 'informed' choices about and to give 'informed' consent for treatment options, which they have been advised. Patient education is the final common pathway and thus a critical requirement for patients to successfully manage their disease. Information is a form of therapy and should lead to more realistic outcome expectations, better treatment compliance and better outcomes. It also allows the patient to be much more involved with the care. As the medical profession changes from a paternalistic (I know what is best for you) model to a patient choice model, patient education will take on a much greater role. It is through patients' as well as their care providers' needs to learn that can play such a vital role on the threshold of this new and exciting era.

Education helps to build a partnership for disease management. Rigorous studies have documented the importance of patient education and communication in all components of clinical care. To manage asthma, for instance, patients might need to carry out complex medication plans, initiate home environmental changes, monitor asthma symptoms and coordinate care between different healthcare providers. The National Heart, Lung and Blood Institute (NHLBI) guidelines recommend that clinicians teach patients these essential skills, and integrate and reinforce patient education into every step of clinical care. The questions we now face are how to efficiently and cost-effectively incorporate education into practice, how to use new technologies and how to offer such education in a culturally competent manner. Both IT and nurses (with special training in communication skills) have great potential in meeting this challenge.

DECISION AIDS FOR PATIENTS

Decision aids for a variety of health conditions are available to help patients take an active and informed role in health decision-making by providing understandable information about treatment options and the individual risks, harms and realistic expectations of possible health outcomes (expressed with probabilities and uncertainties). By using evidence-based medicine and sophisticated risk statistics, patients can be informed [often with clever visual diagrams, videos or compact disk, read only memory (CD-ROM)] and given the opportunity to align their personal values, and arrive at a decision, i.e. best suited for their health status and preferences. These tools can aid in patient counseling and guiding patients in the collaborative decision-making process.

A Cochrane review noted that the availability of the decision aids is expanding with many on the internet; however, few of these have been evaluated. Trials indicate that the decision aids improve knowledge and realistic expectations; enhance active participation in decision-making; lower decisional conflicts; decrease the proportion of people remaining undecided and improve agreement between the value and the choice. Thus, computers and the internet-based resources are unarguably among the optimal strategies for the dissemination of patient and parent education.

PATIENT INFORMATION-SEEKING BEHAVIOR IN THE IT AGE

According to a United States (US) study, 62% of internet users (73 million adults) search for healthcare information. The average user starts at a search site, visits between two and five different health sites, and spent at least 30 minutes on a particular search. Most people look for information about a specific condition that affects them or someone they know; 55% gathered information on the internet before visiting their physicians.

In another study, 72% of respondents reported that health information was easy to find; 85% thought it easy to understand; 82% found it to be of good quality and 93% believed the information to be trustworthy. Furthermore, 30% noted that the information influenced their discussions with their physicians and 17% admitted that the information affected how they would comply with treatment.

Given that many patients research their conditions online, healthcare providers must be aware that patients may have developed preconceived notions about their diagnoses and management before ever seeing their physician. Not all patients come to the office with stacks of printouts or even admit that they have researched their condition. However, the current trend has altered the role of the clinician from keeper of information to interpreter and integrator of information for patients. Thus, instead of being the authoritative information source that they were in the past, physicians today must help patients interpret information that they have gathered, guide them to reliable sources of information and develop a strategy for finding, and integrating new information. The failure of a physician to remain open-minded about such information can lead to frustration for both the patient and the physician. Looking at what a patient has found is helpful in determining whether it is credible and applicable to the patient's specific situation. Patients usually appreciate being redirected to authentic and relevant information. This is where nurses can play a key role.

There are many free resources to which the physicians and the nurses can direct their patients for more information. Links or web addresses can be incorporated into a website, handouts and Android applications. This provides the opportunity for healthcare providers to guide patients toward credible and updated medical information.

EVALUATING THE QUALITY OF INTERNET HEALTH INFORMATION CONTENT

The World Wide Web (www) offers new, inexpensive and rapid methods to provide and enhance patient education. Unlike traditional patient handouts, the internet offers user interactivity and engagement, which should enhance user learning and understanding. However, although patient education websites are widespread, a comprehensive survey of such websites for asthma noted that such information is 'highly variable in quality and content, and makes little innovative use of technology'. No mechanism, however, exists for policing the accuracy of this information.

The internet, now an increasingly pervasive part of our culture, has vastly increased the rate at which information is disseminated. Unfortunately, a substantial portion of the available medical information is incorrect or misleading. Realizing this, many patients would like their physicians to help guide their online searches for medical information. In recommending medical websites, healthcare providers need to consider the quality of the website, the quality of the content and especially the ethics of the site. The most important ethical standard a website must meet is the clear separation of its editorial comment from promotional material. Patients do not have enough knowledge to distinguish unbiased information from information designed to push a product or service. There are organizations such as the Health on the Net Foundation (HON) and the e-Health Code of Ethics that have established clear quality and ethical criteria, but very few resources exist for these organizations to use in policing the sites that claim to adhere to their criteria. Healthcare providers can use these criteria, e.g. from http://www.hon.ch/HONcode/Conduct.html to evaluate the quality of patient education websites and help patients improve their online 'searches' for health information. Perceiving the individual—at times, unique needs of patients, nurses can guide them to websites selected in this manner.

The National Institutes of Health has started a consumer website (www.medlineplus.gov) that takes websites that adhere to their stringent criteria and places them on their website, thus ensuring proper compliance.

Preparing Patients for the Office Visit

Well-designed educational resources and tools can also help patients learn more effective communication skills for the healthcare setting, prepare for their visits by organizing their thoughts and notes, and build awareness with educational materials that facilitate a more informed interaction to occur at the time of an office visit. When patients have considered the medical issues ahead of time, they may be more likely to ask pertinent questions and effectively partner in decision-making. Enhanced patient readiness for an office visit may also yield dividends in terms of what is accomplished, how efficiently it is accomplished and how satisfied the patient is. The pressures of limited time for office appointments and the questionable retention of information following a single interview can also be thus addressed.

In the Doctor's Office

Guidelines recommend that patients, especially those suffering from chronic diseases, receive a written action plan that includes overall goals of therapy, doses and frequencies of medications, and actions to take in the event of an exacerbation or an emergency. Here IT can complement the roles of the physician and the nurse. Well-designed patient handouts with relevant information and instructions are an important and effective means of communication. These reinforce the advice given in the personal interview and provide a written record for review by the patient when in doubt. Charts to be maintained by the patient, e.g. a home blood sugar monitoring with diet chart for a diabetic can be generated, customized and demonstrated using a computer. Showing visuals of diabetic foot or diabetic retinopathy is a sure shot way to improve compliance to therapy. Most patients would welcome a CD-ROM with anticipatory guidance for prevention of complications and advice on injection technique, home-monitoring and general care. Excellent patient handouts are available to doctors from the subscription-based website (www.mdconsult.com). There are a number of websites that continue to provide health education material free of cost.

A patient education process that includes videos may alleviate emotional and physical difficulties lung cancer patients face before and after an operation, according to a new study published in the Journal of the American College of Surgeons. Researchers developed a 30-minute video that offered information on the entire lung operation experience, including what should happen each day after surgery until discharge and what to expect several months later. The video also covered pain management issues and provided information on warning signs for possible problems following discharge and where patients should go for help.

Information technology-enabled patient education resources are a veritable boon for families with a case of rare disease, e.g. inborn errors of metabolism, rare forms of complex structural heart disease and the like. At the tips of ones fingers, one can summon useful information even in remote areas, where local medical expertise and experience may be limited. Besides, taking a second opinion in tricky cases is a time-honored practice and its merits are appreciated by both the patient and the doctor. In today's world, IT-based patient education can sometimes serve this function and simplify decision-making on the patient's part.

Online Support Groups

Support group and online-community sites exist for many disorders and can be an excellent resource for patients because they can interact anonymously at their convenience with others, who have similar problems. These sites host useful links, news updates and dedicated chat rooms in addition to providing general information on the topic of interest. Many patient-support groups have e-mail based discussions that are archived on the web. These are a great boon especially when rare disorders are concerned; information is a very valuable commodity in such cases and communication by any other means may just not be feasible when the correspondents are separated geographically.

Online groups could also be a source of great solace and motivation to the families of differently abled individuals and even to patients fighting cancer or persons living with acquired immunodeficiency syndrome (AIDS). These could provide a platform for sharing experiences and still maintaining privacy. Nuggets of precious information could be exchanged between individuals from around the world. Alternatively, for some groups, such as adolescents with diabetes or asthma, peer groups can be an important social influence that shapes behavior and can be used to help facilitate improved understanding and management of the disease. Due to the complexities of the disease processes in the genetic and chronic diseases, support groups form an integral part of the long-term management of these conditions. Several of the online resources from all around the world offer a variety of services that include educational materials, consultations, group therapy, team building activities and other resources to teach individuals how to cope and adapt to the lifestyle that is often dictated by their illnesses. Few of these are from WHO support group, genomics and disease prevention, Centers for Disease Control Prevention (CDC), Genetic Interest Group (UK) and Medivision India.

Adolescent Counseling

The area where the matchless potential of information technology to facilitate patient (client) education could be harnessed to utmost benefit is reproductive health education and family life counseling of adolescents. Teens are often reluctant to select brochures or handouts with sensitive topics because they do not wish their parents, adults or other patients in the waiting room to see, which pamphlets they select. On the other hand, this technology-savvy subset of healthcare clients and their parents would appreciate anonymous access to reliable yet simple information from responsible professionals on issues ranging from adolescent sexuality to contraception to sexually transmitted diseases (STD). This would help avoid many an embarrassing situation and also go a long way in preventing the tragic consequences of lack of knowledge of the basic facts of life among adolescents.

Many excellent videos are available in the areas of contraception, contraceptive compliance, sexuality, menstrual hygiene, and even anger resolution and conflict management within relationships. Setting aside a small room for patient viewing with a selection of videos available may facilitate the conversations that are initiated by the healthcare provider. Teens also do not like to be lectured and a patronizing or judgmental tone can put them off. Application of IT could be the 'cool' answer to this dilemma. As many teens have access to computers at home, a listing of helpful websites may also serve to emphasize information provided in the office. This approach has the additional great advantage of being non-directive and non-threatening (Box 14.1).

Box 14.1: Advantages of information technology (IT)-assisted patient education

- Information available anytime, anywhere
- Exhaustive coverage in compact form
- Searching for relevant information by preferences easy
- Can be made interactive
- Can be easily updated
- Persistence of message for repeated access
- Multimedia permits extensive use of images, audio and video
- May have greater appeal and impact than conventional means
- No geographical barriers
- Can be stored indefinitely without space constraints or clutter

Correspondence

E-mail is a convenient way of communicating with patients and it's anytime-anywhere accessibility is a great boon. Although, corresponding with patients via E-mail is easy, there are many issues to consider; the biggest well-founded concerns are related to confidentiality and liability, especially if ground rules are not established between patients and physicians. Besides, an increasing and universal use of smart phones and mobile applications are now viewed as a boon to the outreach of medical information and technology, and hence the utility of E-mail as a tool for patient education and information is going to be further limited.

Some Useful Patient Resources

Some medical journals feature patient information pages on the internet, such as the Journal of the American Medical Association (http://www.jama.com/), Annals of Internal Medicine (http://www.annals.org/), Postgraduate Medicine (http://www.postgradmed.com/) and Patient Care (http://www.patientcareonline.com/). The National Women's Health Resource Center covers consumer educational needs for a variety of topics in women's health (http://www.healthywomen.org/). Other websites, such as MerckMedicus (http://www.merckmedicus.com/) integrate a variety of healthcare resources, providing clinicians with access to resources, such as medical textbooks, journals and up-to-date news clips. The accompanying patient-friendly site called MerckSource (http://www.mercksource.com/) features printable descriptions of medical conditions, lifestyle advice and other educational resources to empower patients to participate in their own care, and decision-making.

Over 500 patient education topics also can be viewed at and printed from the free site sponsored by the American Academy of Family Physicians (http://www.familydoctor.org). The American Medical Association (http://www.ama-assn.org/) has extensive patient-education materials (http://www.ama-assn.org/sitemap.htm/consumer) is a list of websites posted by the American Medical Association.

The American Academy of Otolaryngology—Head and Neck Surgery has a page for patients that describe how to find reliable health information on the Internet (http://www.entlink.net/healthinfo/about/reliable ent.cfm). There are also sites that allow patients to rate their individual providers and healthcare facilities (e.g. http://www.healthgrades.com/).

Local Patient Education Resources

Practices and institutions could incorporate education resources into their websites for their patients to access uploaded information form. A pediatric practice, could have web pages with information on vaccination schedules, infant feeding, growth and development, accident prevention, first aid for common emergencies, etc. Needless to add, these require being updated and improved regularly with due attention to accessibility, accuracy, appropriateness and appeal. Nurses can help patients find their way in this maze of health information. Hosting a Frequently Asked Questions (FAQs) page is a popular way of getting messages across in a user-friendly format.

There might be discordance of messages that are received from the variety of providers a patient might see in different settings. Sharing of professionally authenticated education resources via internet links can ensure that the messages from different sources are consistent and reinforce each other. Physicians and nurses will need to focus on their role as counselors to prevent the emergence of 'cyberchondriacs.'

A recent review provides evidence that multimedia education about medications is more effective than usual care (non-standardized education provided by health professionals as part of usual clinical care) or no education, in improving both knowledge and skill acquisition. It also suggests that multimedia education is at least equivalent to other forms of education, including written education and education provided by a health professional. However, this finding is based on often low-quality evidence from a small number of trials. Multimedia education about medications could therefore be considered as an adjunct to usual care, but there is inadequate evidence to recommend it as a replacement for written education or education by a health professional.

INDIA: THE GROUND REALITIES AND FUTURE POSSIBILITIES

In India, with illiteracy and language differences being a barrier, the use of images can be effective in conveying messages through an audiovisual medium for powerful impact. With IT, it is also possible to adapt the same patient educational material with script and commentary in several languages. This simple measure will ensure that no patient is denied the benefits of education. With all schools, even those in the remotest areas, set to get access to computers, it would not be too ambitious to envisage a scenario, where all health facilities too would be equipped similarly. Satellite technology to provide access to the internet, though prohibitively expensive in the short term, may yield rich dividends in the long run. This may be one solution for reaching the unreached in our country's vast geographical expanse. Just as people have become comfortable banking and making purchases online, they will come to expect more complex IT-assisted or online interactions with their healthcare providers.

NURSES: POTENTIAL TECHNOLOGY SAVVY PATIENT EDUCATORS

Nursing is a holistic discipline. Since the days of Florence Nightingale, nursing has been associated with warmth and caring. Now, the 'information explosion' is set to add a new dimension to the role of nurses. In addition to carrying out 'routine' duties pertaining to daily patient care, nurses have always been involved in patient (and caretaker) education, counseling, support and rehabilitation. Nurses are at an advantageous position when it comes to their role as professionals imparting patient education on healthcare issues.

A patient can relate much more easily and directly to the nurse than perhaps to the doctor, and importantly the nurse can devote the time required to give individualized information and guidance. The element of the personal human touch might determine patient compliance.

In the patient's perception, the nurse is the right mix of the professional and the lay. Information and education are among the key expectations of patients from their care-providers and often it is these aspects that decide whether or not the patient returns. After the principal clinician introduces key messages, different members of the healthcare team should reinforce and expand these messages during office visits and telephone calls or in more formal education sessions, e.g. in a group education session in a diabetes clinic.

NURSING INFORMATICS

The term, 'nursing informatics' was probably first used by Scholes and Barber in 1980, and defined as the application of computer technology to all fields of nursing such as nursing services, nursing education and nursing research. The 2001 American Nursing Association (ANA) definition labels it as a specialty that integrates nursing science, computer science, and information science to manage and communicate data, information and knowledge in nursing practice. Further, nursing informatics facilitates the integration of data, information and knowledge to support patients, nurses and other providers in their decision-making in all roles and settings. This support is accomplished through the use of information structures, information processes and information technology. Patient education is obviously one of the key areas of application.

CONCLUSION

Patient education from sources other than face-to-face contact with a healthcare provider should be seen as a beneficial adjunct to the medical practice of physicians and not as competition. Doctors and nurses will continue to provide the irreplaceable human angle even as information technology enriches the patient-provider interaction. Health consumers increasingly want access to accurate, evidence-based information about their medications. Currently, health education and patient information about medications, i.e. information, which is designed to achieve health or illness-related learning is provided predominantly via spoken communication between the health provider and consumer, sometimes supplemented with written materials. There is some evidence that current educational methods are not meeting consumer needs. Multimedia educational programs offer many potential advantages over traditional forms of education delivery. It is time to embrace the IT age. The tremendous potential for information technology in healthcare is only beginning to be actualized.

FURTHER READING

1. Available from http://www.beckers hospitalreview.com/quality/patient-education [Accessed September 5, 2013].
2. Available from http: www.who.int/genomics/public/patientssuport/en [Accessed August 25, 2013].
3. Available from http://www.mercksource.com/ [Accessed August 28, 2013].
4. Vidyashankar C. Information technology and parent education. Asian J Pediatr Practice. 2004;8:55-8.

15

Hospital Information Systems

Jagdish Chinnappa

Hospital information systems (HIS) are computer-based software applications that integrate many medical, nursing, administrative and miscellaneous functions of a healthcare set up. All information systems that enhance patient care in hospitals would contribute to a HIS. These software packages vary from simple applications to very complex ones, depending on the goals and the endpoints defined by the hospitals.

There are two main aspects of the HIS, the front end and the back end. The front-end functions include patient care, administrative functions, financial components, research and training, while the back-end functions include the hardware, software and the information technology (IT) support staff.

FRONT-END FUNCTIONS

Patient Care

Electronic Medical Record

The most important of HIS will be to ensure smooth and efficient management of the patient, and reduction in errors that are very common in big hospitals essentially due to the complexity of care involved. When a patient enters a hospital, the starting point is scheduling appointments. With an efficient HIS, appointment scheduling is extremely efficient. Patients can get appointments at short notice and any delays can be confirmed via short message service (SMS) or e-mail. As soon as the patient needs to be admitted in hospital, registration and identification through a unique code is done. This is vital to protect the confidentiality of the patient and insurance formalities. Once admitted, the patient can be shifted to an appropriate area, bed vacancy and availability are easily discernible with the help of HIS.

Appropriate medical and nursing plans can be initiated, which will be documented on the hospital information systems. Alerts for allergies and drug interactions can be immediately recognized. Medication ordering and administration at appropriate times can be achieved through HIS. Any allergies that the patient may have can be entered into the system and this will ensure enhanced safety for the patient.

Care must be taken that the accredited physician authorizes medication orders. These are called physician order entry (POE). The medication list can also be transmitted to the pharmacy for appropriate action. Scheduling procedures in the intensive care unit (ICU) and in the operation theater becomes easier when an efficient HIS is in place. Investigations, both laboratory and radiology can be scheduled efficiently with HIS. Logistic planning in terms of transport and care of the patient during and after the procedure is important to ensure patient comfort. Most hospitals have HIS systems that will support the viewing of laboratory report and alerts at the patient's bedside. Images can also be used at the patient's bedside through sophisticated system like picture archiving and communication system (PACS). Clinical workflow decisions over time can be planned. Transferring the patient to specialized areas like ICU is also very easily done using HIS.

Coding for the patient's illness is a very important part of management. This is because most billing procedures are linked to coding. Insurance reimbursement is also a vital part dependent of coding. Administration of nutrition and fluids require smooth collaboration with the hospital dietetic department. It is very important that this department also has a competent information system. Discharge procedures of the patient would need a thorough medical and nursing summary. Follow-up actions once the patient is discharged can also be scheduled with HIS.

One of the most important part of the HIS is communication amongst all the caregivers. Usually every patient has multiple doctors and nurses, and other paramedical staff caring for him/her, unless there is proper communication amongst all these caregivers there is always a scope for errors. A properly functioning HIS will eliminate the number of errors. In addition to the general HIS, there may be specialized packages for different specialties like neonatology or oncology. The typical fields in an electronic medical record are shown in Box 15.1.

Administrative Functions

Running a hospital involves high quality administrative function. Some of the key functions, which can be easily managed with the HIS, are as follows.

Box 15.1: An example of electronic medical record

- Allergies and alerts
- Chief complaints
- Current illness
- Physical measurements
- Family, social and medical history
- Patient own medication
- Clinical notes
- Questionnaire
- Floor plan notes
- Scan/Upload documents
- Image annotation
- Observations
- Results
- Medication orders

Facility Management

Taking care of the infrastructure of the hospital building in terms of cleanliness, lightings, lifts, toilets, corridors, water, electricity and security systems is a big challenge that has to be executed on a daily basis. Proper systems can be set up using HIS.

Human Resource Development

In a hospital, there are a large number of employees working at different levels, medical, paramedical and nonmedical. It is very important that proper systems are in place to take care of these employees.

Medical Records Department

Maintaining medical records and archiving is extremely important, both from the medicolegal angle and for the care of the patient. Stringent systems will be necessary to maintain patient confidentiality.

Maintaining Stock and Store Management

In a hospital, a large inventory of drugs, devices and instruments need to be kept at proper management of the stock is vital to ensure availability and to reduce redundancy.

Other Functions

Some of the other administrative functions, which are very important are waste disposal, catering, security, policy as far as visitors are concerned, quality management and adhering to international standards.

Financial

One of the main functions of HIS is proper billing and recovery of accounts. Financial accounting is very important. Other functions of the financial system could be cost accounting, resource allocation and long-term financial planning.

Research

Most big hospitals are involved in clinical trials. It is very important that these trials are within the ambit of the regulatory authority. An efficient HIS will help right through the process of clinical trials. Well-implemented HIS will be invaluable in retrieving retrospective data for publication and for looking at trends of diseases.

Teaching

Health information system can be used for teaching and training, personnel at all levels. Telemedicine can be used for remote teaching, training, second opinions and consultations.

BACK-END FUNCTIONS

Implementation of the HIS

To implement a HIS from a large bouquet of available systems needs an experienced medical information team. They should study the needs of the institution and plan for the future growth of the institution. The HIS should be both cost and time effective. Training personnel to use the system should be simple and scalable. Some of the key components are:

- Hardware
- Software
- Connectivity
- Data storage
- Peripherals
- Power backup
- Availability on portable systems.

Hardware

Hardware usually consists of a server stored in a secure place and multiple terminals at individual sites. The heart of the hardware is a powerful network server (NS). This NS offers a centralized location and software installation for multiple functions. The NS can be a single point for upgrades backup, print, email and many other functions. Terminals situated at workstations are connected to the NS by cables.

For the user, terminal to access software resides in the NS, permission in the form of passwords are needed. Depending upon the hierarchy in the hospital, access could be given to only some parts of the information stored in the NS. The NS is protected physically by temperature and other environmental safeguards.

Cloud Storage

Future is the cloud: Many organizations are moving from NS to cloud computing. Here the access to software and storage of data is done on remote locations using the internet. While there may be advantages of cost and convenience, there are issues that need to be resolved before it can become popular for HIS. The main concern is of confidentiality.

Software

The NS needs to have an array of software programs, which must be integrated. Some of these are:

1. Database management: Oracle, structured query language (SQL), uniplexed information and computer systems (UNIX), access.
2. Antivirus: McAfee, Norton, QuickHeal.
3. Client-server technology software: CORBAmed.
4. Image management: Pacs.
5. Voice recognition: Dragon.
6. Medical decision-making.
7. Peripherals: Printers, scanners software.
8. Internet.
9. Statistics.
10. Office software: Word, Excel and PowerPoint.

Connectivity (Network)

All the terminals need to be connected to the NS. This is done through standard cabling.

Data Storage

1. The data captured in the hospital has to be reliably stored.
2. Hospitals spend huge amounts of money for secure storage of data.
3. This is extremely important to safeguard the confidentiality of the patient.
4. Data storage guidelines have been recently released by the Government of India.

Peripherals

Peripherals are devices that are connected to terminals. They include printers, scanners, cameras bar code machines and many others. The type of peripherals depends on the nature of data capture and output that is needed. Software for these peripherals could be located in the terminals or the network server.

Power Backup

Health information system should have an uninterrupted non-fluctuant supply of electricity. Backup uninterrupted power supply (UPS) systems and generators are vital. Any interruption of power and power surges can lead to loss of precious data.

Availability on Portable Systems

Tablets and handheld devices have invaded the market. Their sleekness and portability have allowed electronic medical records (EMRs) to be instilled in them. They can be carried to the patient's bedside and can be connected by wireless networks. There may be some compromise on functionality.

CONCLUSION

Hospital information systems (HIS) are row becoming important tools in the functioning of the health care set ups. Their benefits would ensure efficient management of the patients with their records and also an improved administrative functioning.

FURTHER READING

1. Available from http://www.emrconsultant.com/emr-education-center/emr-selection-his [Accessed on November 10, 2014].
2. Jahanbakhsh M, Sharifi M, Ayat M. The status of hospital information systems in Iranian hospitals. Acta Inform Med. 2014;22(4):268-75.

16

Statistical Packages: Types and their Features

Nishtha Kathuria Juneja, Sumeet Juneja

INTRODUCTION

'Statistics' can simply mean something expressed in numbers. Different authors have defined statistics differently. The best definition of statistics is given by Croxton and Cowden according to whom statistics may be defined as the science, which deals with collection, presentation, analysis and interpretation of numerical data.[1]

For example *your hospital has 5000 OPD admissions per year. The average length of stay is 3 days. Over 60% of nurses are trained in critical care.*

This chapter deals with basics of statistics in brief, need of statistics for nurses and statistical packages commonly used.

You probably make statistical statements in your everyday conversation or thinking, even though you may not realize. Statements like 'I sleep for about eight hours per night on average' and 'You are more likely to pass the exam if you start preparing earlier' are actually statistical in nature.

Today, statistics has become an important tool in the work of many academic disciplines such as medicine, psychology, education, sociology, engineering and physics, just to name a few. Statistics is also important in many aspects of society such as business, industry and government. Because of the increasing use of statistics in so many areas of our lives, it has become very desirable to understand and practise statistical thinking.

ROLE OF STATISTICS IN NURSING

Nurses use statistics in day to day functioning and need to have a working understanding of it, if not detailed knowledge. Some common examples of day to day applications of statistics in nursing are the number of occupied beds in each ward daily, the number of patients with special nutritional needs measurement of improvement indicators (to determine the progress made), etc.

Florence Nightingale is the first known nurse statistician. She used statistical techniques to prove the effectiveness of sanitary conditions (simple things like sunshine, fresh air, clean dressing, etc.) in preventing military deaths.

Statistical results are very useful to show a trend, rather than relying on emotional appeals. For example, instead of saying that nurses are over-worked, we can simply state the statistics and show that for every extra patient load on a nurse, chances of death increase by 7%. In simpler terms, more nurses mean fewer deaths. Statistics help in patient care and improving the nursing practice. For example, statistics can show the effectiveness of a new practice, say the effect of using a new type of gloves or anti-septic medicine, etc. Statistics help in quantifying phenomena, which is much easier to think about and discuss than qualitative trends.

BROAD CATEGORIES OF STATISTICS

Descriptive statistics: It encompasses the tabular, graphical or pictorial display of data, condensation of large data into tables, preparation of summary measures to give a concise description of complex information and also to exhibit pattern that may be found in data sets.

Inferential statistics: Inferential statistics however refers to decisions.

STATISTICAL PACKAGES

Computer based statistical packages are an important tool for research in the health, education and social sectors. The prospect of using statistics is sometimes frightening for people, yet most researchers recognize the potential utility of statistical analysis to aid them to describe, analyze, interpret and report their data. The packages have reduced the need to be able to undertake many of the calculations that are required for statistical analyses. In this way these packages allow to concentrate on understanding the assumptions behind the various methods, as well as the potential applications and limitations of various statistical tests. More recent computer software packages are reasonably easy to use for people with some familiarity with computers. Most of the packages have features such as drop-down menus, 'tree' structure diagrams and on-line help systems. When choosing which package to use for statistical analyses a number of factors must be considered. These include the availability of a package, its cost, the functions it can perform, familiarity with the package and the availability of an expert statistician to assist with the analysis process.[2]

There are about 50 statistical packages and with advancing technology new packages are being added.

This chapter only describes 3 packages which are relevant for nurses.

Epi Info[3]

Epi Info is a package which is most suitable for doctors and researchers. It is a package which suffices for nearly all the usual clinical research and epidemiological settings. Epi Info is a public domain database and statistics program for performing statistical applications in clinical research. Statistics, graphs, tables, and maps can be produced with simple commands. Epi Info is free, downloadable software provided by the CDC (www.cdc.gov/epiinfo/) and has been developed as a joint collaboration between WHO and CDC, Atlanta.

Epi Info™ is a public domain suite of interoperable software tools designed for the global community of public health practitioners and researchers. It provides for easy data entry form and database construction, a customized data entry experience, and data analyses with epidemiologic statistics, maps, and graphs for public health professionals who may lack an information technology background. Epi Info™ is used for outbreak investigations; for developing small to mid-sized disease surveillance systems; as analysis, visualization, and reporting (AVR) components of larger systems; and in the continuing education in the science of epidemiology and public health analytic methods at schools of public health around the world.

Latest epi Info is available for windows, mobiles and web and cloud.

How to Download

1. Go to www.cdc.gov/**epiinfo**
2. Download installer
3. Follow instructions on screen
4. Open desktop shortcut

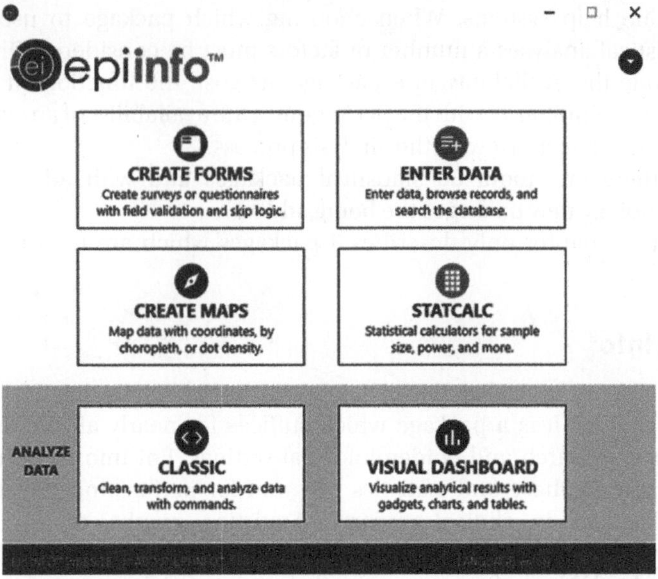

Epi Info™ 7 is comprised of four main tools used to collect, analyze, or visualize data:

1. **Create forms:** Create a questionnaire using one or more forms to collect and view data.
2. **Enter Data:** Enter data and view existing records.
3. **Analyze Data (Classic and Visual Dashboard):** Manage data, run statistical analyses, and generate lists, tables, graphs, and charts.
4. **Create Maps:** Create maps from map server, KLM files, or shape files.

Available utilities include:

1. **StatCalc:** Compute statistics from summary data.
2. **Help:** Find online and offline resources: including a 'discussion forum'
3. 'help desk' information.
4. **Options:** Configure default settings on the following tabs: general, language, analysis, plug-ins, and web survey.

MS EXCEL

Excel is probably the most commonly used spreadsheet for PCs. Newly purchased computers often arrive with Excel already loaded.

It is easily used to do a variety of calculations, includes a collection of statistical functions, and a Data Analysis ToolPak. The advantages include:

- Nearly ubiquitous and is often pre-installed on new computers
- User friendly
- Very good for basic descriptive statistics, charts and plots.

Managing and Tabulating Data in Excel

Rows and columns are used for tabulating the data. Click on cell A1 and enter the first number in the set of numbers that you are investigating. Press 'Enter' and the program will automatically select cell A2 for you. Enter the second number into cell A2 and continue until you have entered the entire set of numbers into column A.

S.No	Patient Name	Age	Sex	Hb (in gm/dl)
1	Pankaj	23	M	12.2
2	Jia	30	F	14
3	Nikita	34	F	13.2
4	Balpreet	34	M	13.4
5	Upant	25	M	11.6
6	Hemant	45	M	9.4
7	Garima	16	F	7.3
8	Sanjay	23	M	10.4
9	Manish	27	M	11.7
10	Shivani	29	F	10.3
11	Irfan	36	M	9.9
12	Aasim	38	M	11.3
13	Roza	46	F	12
14	Faiyaz	41	M	13.6
15	Bhupesh	30	M	14.2

Functions

1. **Calculate mean:** Click on cell. Enter the following formula, without quotes, to find the arithmetic mean of your set of numbers: '=AVERAGE (Insert range)'. Press 'Enter' to complete the formula and the mean of your numbers will appear in the cell.

In the above mentioned, e.g. mean of Hb would be '=average(E2:E16)'

2. **Calculate median:** Enter the following formula, without quotes, into the cell: '=MEDIAN(A:A)'. Press 'Enter' and the median of your set of numbers will appear in the cell.

   In the above mentioned, e.g. mean of Hb would be '=mean(E2:E16)'

3. **Calculate mode:** Click cell where you wish to calculate mode. Enter the following formula, without quotes, into the cell: '=MODE.MULT(A:A)'. Press 'Enter' and the cell will display mode of the data set.
4. **Calculate range:** Select cell. Enter the following formula, without quotes, into the cell: '=MAX(A:A)-MIN(A:A)'. Press 'Enter' and the cell will display the range for your set of data.
5. **Calculate standard deviation:** Select cell . Enter the following formula, without quotes, into the cell: '=STDEV(A:A)'. Press 'Enter' and the cell will display the range for your set of data.

Making Charts

Step 1: Select data

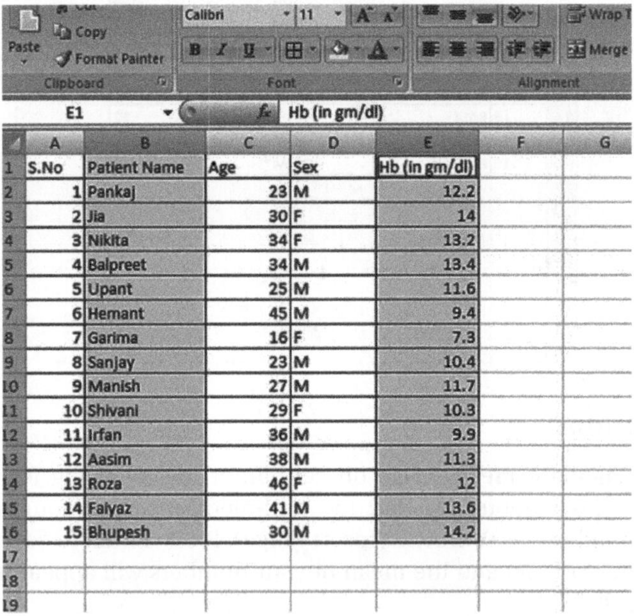

S.No	Patient Name	Age	Sex	Hb (in gm/dl)
1	Pankaj	23	M	12.2
2	Jia	30	F	14
3	Nikita	34	F	13.2
4	Balpreet	34	M	13.4
5	Upant	25	M	11.6
6	Hemant	45	M	9.4
7	Garima	16	F	7.3
8	Sanjay	23	M	10.4
9	Manish	27	M	11.7
10	Shivani	29	F	10.3
11	Irfan	36	M	9.9
12	Aasim	38	M	11.3
13	Roza	46	F	12
14	Faiyaz	41	M	13.6
15	Bhupesh	30	M	14.2

Step 2: Insert chart

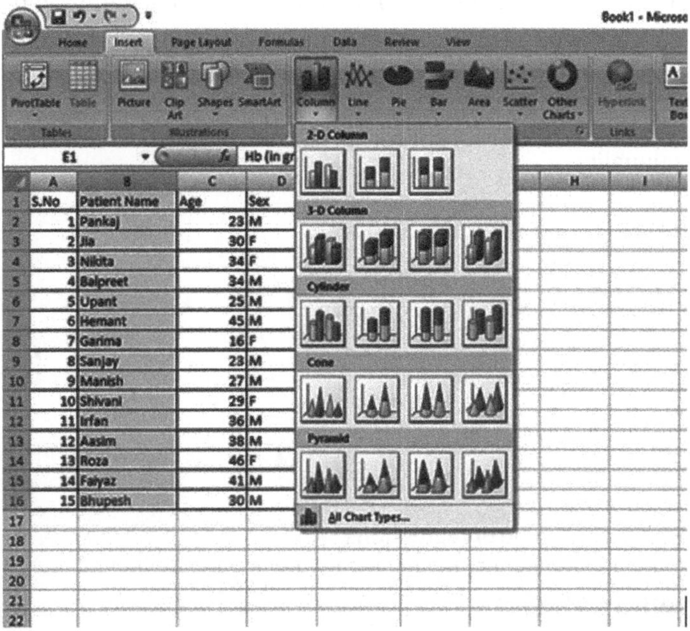

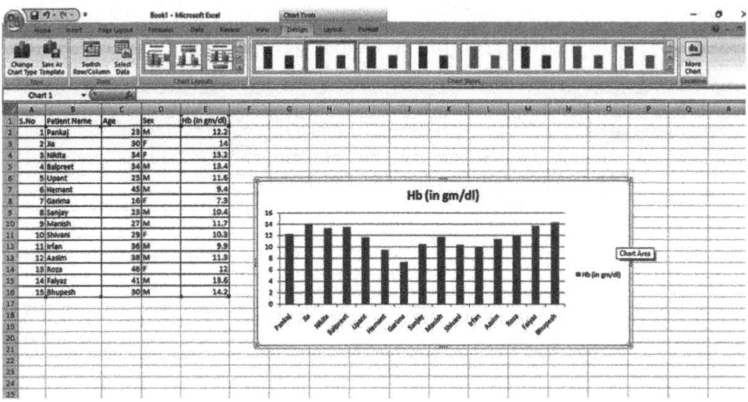

STATISTICAL PACKAGE FOR SOCIAL SCIENCES (SPSS)

The Statistical Package for the Social Sciences (SPSS) is a widely used program for statistical analysis in social sciences, particularly in education and research. However, because of its potential, it is also widely used by market researchers, health care researchers, survey organizations, governments and, most notably, data miners and big data professionals.[2]

It is presently one of the most commonly used statistical packages research institutions. The advantages of the package are its relative ease of use, its familiarity to many statistical experts and its functionality.

What can You do with SPSS?

- Run frequencies
- Calculate descriptive statistics
- Compare means
- Conduct cross-tabulations
- Recode data
- Create graphs and charts
- Do T-Tests
- Conduct ANOVAs
- Run various type of regressions

Opening SPSS

When you open SPSS, a data window will open at the bottom are two tabs (see at the bottom left of the image below):

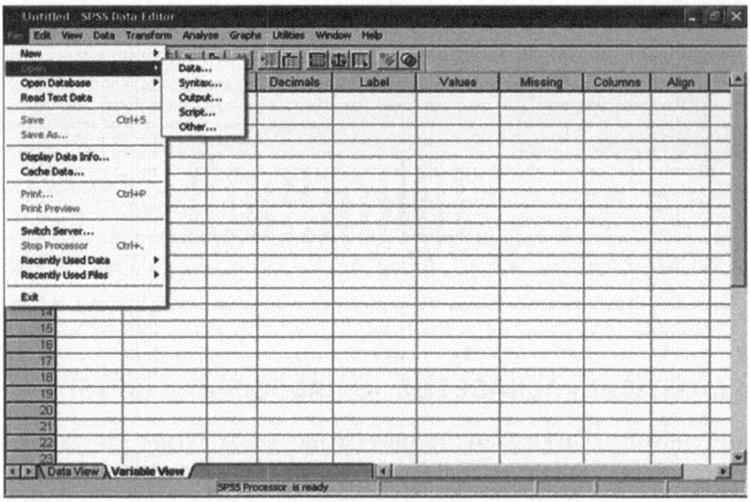

- **Data view:** Gives title of each variable at top, and allows you to enter your data, case by case
- **Variable view:** Gives the details of each variables, and allows you to define/describe the variables in your research.

SPSS has Three Parts/Windows

- **Data:** Where you enter the data (.sav)
- **Syntax:** Where details of the analyses you are going to do are displayed (.sps)
- **Viewer/Output:** Where the results are displayed (.spo)—any messages (such as errors) are displayed in this window.
  You must always have a data window open, and you do not have to use the syntax window—if an output window is open, messages appear in this, and it remains where it was (e.g. behind the data screen).

Using SPSS

This involves three steps:

1. Set up data sheet
2. Enter data
3. Run analyses

There are many more options in the menus, for example:

- **Transpose:** New data file switching cases/variables
- **Merge files:** Combines two data files
- **Aggregate:** Combine cases/variables in a new data file
- **Split files:** Look at results breaking down by variables
- **Select cases:** Choose only certain cases and then run analyses on these.

SUMMARY

Medical and paramedical researchers frequently collect large quantities of data, from surveys, experiments and other forms of observation. A statistical computing package provides a convenient means to store these data, and derive descriptive and inferential statistics. The statistical packages described in this chapter are widely used general-purpose survey analysis package, and hence a useful one to master. It is necessary to allow some learning time to become familiar with this package.

ENDNOTES

1. Agarwal S, Basannar DR, Bhalwar R et al., Textbook of Public Health and Community Medicine, Pune, 2008.
2. Emtage, Nick F and Duthy, Stephen (2002). An Introduction to Statistical Package for the Social Sciences. In: Harrison, Steve R, Herbohn, John L, Mangaoang, Eduardo O and Vanclay, Jerome K, *Socio-Economic Research Methods in Forestry: A Training Manual*, Leyte State University, ViSCA, Baybay, The Philippines, (53-64). 4-10 February, 2002.
3. https://www.cdc.gov/epiinfo/index.html

17

Telemedicine

Naveen Thacker, Sandeep Thacker

INTRODUCTION

Telemedicine has been defined as the use of telecommunications to provide the medical information and services. To put it simply, telemedicine is the exchange of medical information over a distance. This applies to discussions, images, laboratory data and any other part of medically relevant information. The need for telemedicine arises due to the fact, good quality, accessible, affordable health care is still not available to a large part of Indian population. Deaths in rural areas occur today also due to lack of expert doctors, which can be overcome with the use of telemedicine. It takes experts of health care to the village level and provides people with better health care. A formal definition of telemedicine states that "the use of medical information exchanged from one site to another via electronic communication for the health and education of the patient or healthcare provider, and for the purpose of improving patient care" (The American Telemedicine Association).

It can be as simple as two health professionals discussing a case over telephone or as smart as using satellite technology to broadcast a consultation between facilities in two countries using videoconferencing equipment. Initially, it was restricted to transmitting patient images using TV cameras, which was used at sea, airlines and in remote areas. But, the advent of computers and internet has made the transmission of complete patient data possible. Telemedicine has not only made medical care more accessible in developed countries but it has also helped in providing specialized care in developing countries with the minimal cost.

HISTORY

University of Nebraska did first documented use of visual telecommunication in health care in 1959. Under first international telemedicine program in December 1988, the site of a massive earthquakeinArmeniawaslinkedtomedicalcentersinUnitedStatesfor telemedicine consultations. The program was extended to Russia to provide telemedicine consultation to burn victims after a terrible train accident.

First internet-based telemedicine trial was conducted in April 1995. When a Chinese student Zee Ling who was studying in Beijing University felt sick and her condition could not be diagnosed in China. Some of her friends put all her records on internet. She was diagnosed to have thallium poisoning through internet and she was prescribed treatment through internet.

Telemedicine had made great advancements, since then and today we find in market many blood sugar testing devices, which directly send the results to the doctor's email.

SCOPE OF TELEMEDICINE

Telemedicine not only provides consultation but also education, monitoring and more. Telemedicine falls in four categories:

1. Teleconsultation.
2. Tele-education.
3. Telemonitoring.
4. Telesurgery.

Teleconsultation

As the name suggests, it is the most important component. A doctor or a paramedical health worker in a remote area can have a consultation with a specialist. This requires certain procedures to be followed, the person initiating the request needs to be trained and more importantly the complete process needs to be documented for the patients and the doctor's record. Teleconsultation also involves a family doctor seeking help of specialist in an emergency or otherwise. It also involves getting radiological or pathological opinions from the best specialists.

Teleeducation

Information to the community at large, i.e. teleinformation, on health issues has also been made possible with telemedicine technologies. Internet and satellite communications are now increasingly used as a tool for tele-education, meetings, clinical consultations and video conferencing for surgeries.

Telemonitoring

Telemonitoring is the remote monitoring of patient data. The patient's status can be monitored wherever he/she is whether in an aircraft or in remote village as long he/she has a telephone/internet access. The data includes blood pressure, pulse, electrocardiogram (ECG), spirometry, ultrasound, computed tomography (CT) scan and other radiology data. These can be transmitted using telephone lines or through wireless with the use of appropriate devices that can transmit these data over phone.

Telesurgery

Telesurgery is a technique that enables a surgeon to perform surgery remotely using robotics. All that is required videoconferencing equipment to enable the surgeon to see what they are doing and a communication link to allow the transmission of video to the surgeon and robot commands to the robot, not forgetting the robotic equipment.

ADVANTAGES OF TELEMEDICINE

Resource Utilization

First benefit of telemedicine is proper utilization of resources. In India, doctor population ratio is 1 doctor for every 1,538 persons in comparison to 1 doctor for every 413 persons in United States and these doctors are not distributed equally. Nearly 80% of Indian population lives in rural and semiurban areas. There are few specialists in these areas, while cities are overcrowded with specialists. Telemedicine can help in cost-effective utilization of scanty resources and at the same time can decrease patient workload on few referral centers.

Early Intervention

One of the most effective means of providing medical intervention is by early detection and treatment. In many cases, the initial patient presentation is made in a primary care setting. If the case requires specialty care, an appointment is made for the patient to see a specialist at another time. There are factors that inhibit the continuity of care. Issues such as geographic location, bad weather, socioeconomic barriers and patient's lack of concern are significant factors that delay, and even prevent the specialty care that is required to treat the condition.

By providing these primary care sites with the ability to quickly access specialty consultation services, patients are able to reap the benefits of early intervention, while the healthcare system maintains quality service and clinical efficiency.

Avoids Unnecessary Transportation

Unnecessary referral and patient transport can be definitely avoided. In addition, same telemedicine connection can be used promptly to treat emergencies that may have been undetected.

Community-based Care

Community-based care is additional big advantage of telemedicine. People like to receive high-quality care in their local community. This reduces travel time and related stresses associated with many referrals.

Cost Saving

Technology is becoming increasingly cheaper and the cost of telemedicine has gone down considerably. It has been worked out that telemedicine has resulted in considerable savings more, so in teleradiology and in home care of chronically ill patient. In India, use of telemedicine is expected to reduce the costs considerably. Initial cost for setting up facilities is high, but it reduces costs incurred by the patients and is beneficial in long run.

Improved Patient Documentation

Use of telemedicine ensures that patient data is stored electronically and digitally. This ensures better documentation, which is more accurate and complete.

TYPES OF DATA TRANSFERABLE

Data can be transferred in the form of digital signals. Basically, four types of data are used in telemedicine:

1. Text: For patient notes.
2. Audio: Recorded with help of electronic stethoscope data such as heart sounds, lung sounds, bowel sounds, etc.
3. Still image: X-ray, electrocardiogram (ECG), ultrasound/ CT/magnetic resonance imaging (MRI) and photos of skin conditions or wounds.
4. Video/Movie: Ultrasound/Patient visualization, operative procedures, echocardiogram, angiogram, etc. The patient can be seen by a doctor at a remote place using cameras.

TELEMEDICINE CONCEPTS

Frame Rate and Bandwidth

A video image has a rate of motion knows as the frame rate. This standard video like the one seen on the television has a frame rate of 30 frames per second. This 30 frames per second rate is required, so human eyes does not perceive any gaps in information. In videoconferencing, there is limitation or restriction on the amount of information that can be transmitted through digital lines. This limitation on amount of information that can be transmitted is known as bandwidth. This bandwidth is directly related to cost, more the bandwidth more the cost. To decrease the cost so that less bandwidth is required, video is compressed. As one compresses the video frame rate is decreased. Depending on the available bandwidth, frame rate used may be 7.5, 10, 15 or 30 frames per second. If one uses lower frame rate, picture will appear jumpy or jittery and this is known as motion artifact. If one selects a higher frame rate one has to use more bandwidth. Standard bandwidth used in videoconferencing and telemedicine, range between 64 kbps and 1.544 mbps. Ordinary telephone lines provide maximum bandwidth of 28.8 kbps. Integrated services for digital network (ISDN) lines provide bandwidth of 128 kbps.

Regular telephone lines do not supply adequate bandwidth for most telemedicine applications. For videoconferencing, digital lines are required like ISDN or T1 that are not available in most parts of India.

How this Data can be Transferred?

Digital data can be transferred via ordinary telephone lines [public service telephone network (PSTN)]. Ordinary telephone lines can only transfer analog signal not digital signals. So you need modem at both the places. First modem will convert digital signals to analog signals before sending it through telephone lines. Then at receiving end modem will again convert analog signal to digital signal. This is how data is transferred through telephone lines. Other modes of transferring digital data are digital networks such as ISDN, T1 and asynchronous transfer mode (ATM). All these are very fast, but not available everywhere. Data can also be transferred through internet, intranet, microwave and satellite.

The most important issue in data transmission is bandwidth. For telemedicine, better bandwidth than the PSTN is required to transmit images and audio.

TELEMEDICINE TECHNOLOGIES

There are two types of technology used in telemedicine:

1. Store and forward technology.
2. Real-time telemedicine.

Store and Forward Technology

In store and forward technology, an event is recorded as single image and stored. Then this single image or series of images along with voice, text and data are sent to a specialist through email or modem. This store and forward technology is commonly used in radiology, pathology and dermatology. Most common use of store and forward technology is sending radiological image like CT to a distant specialist and taking their opinion. A drawback of store and forward technology is that it is not interactive, so it cannot be used in emergency situation. Advantages are that cost is less, it can be used using ordinary telephone lines and modem.

Real-time Telemedicine

The telemedicine transaction is processed as soon as it is received. Direct link is established between the remote patient and the health expert. This is of great value in emergencies where store and forward is not useful. This requires real-time equipment and telecommunication facility for transmission of text, images, audio and video images. Videoconferencing is the technology, which is used mostly for real-time telemedicine.

Videoconferencing

Here there are two locations, on one side is patient and local health provider, and on other side is specialist. These two sides are linked by putting videoconferencing instruments at both locations, so a real-time consultation takes place between specialist and patient, and local health provider. Apart from real-time consultation, videoconferencing is also used for real-time teleradiology, where an image is transmitted to a distant radiologist without taking plate, telepathology. Where a intraoperative frozen section may be sent to a distant pathologist from operation theater and course of operation is decided after the report and telerobotic surgery, where a surgeon in one location can remotely control a robotic arm for surgery in another location.

TELEMEDICINE DEVICES

Telemedicine devices are of two types, one for getting the patient information and the other videoconferencing for transmitting it in an unaltered form.

Videoconferencing System

There are various types of videoconferencing systems:

1. Roll about systems: These are movable units comprising a monitor, camera and associated hardware, and can go to any site where it is required.
2. Set top system: These are systems that sit on top of conventional computers and provide the telemedicine service.
3. Desktop systems: The standard personal computer (PC) is modified using PC cards. This is the most economical and also provides the least resolution though with currently available graphic and audiocards, even the ordinary PC can be converted to most powerful telemedicine device with just the addition of a high-resolution camera and ISDN access.

The equipments required for videoconferencing include the following:

1. Digital camera having the zoom and macro facility to access any part of patient and also the facility of videorecording. This needs to be connected to the computer for processing the image using image processing software, which can compress the image and aid in its forward transmission.
2. Audio system with speaker and mike need to be of good quality.

Nowadays, telemedicine software process all the telemedicine input data, and transmit it. All that required is the equipment and the connection to internet.

Peripheral Devices

These are those pieces of equipment or hardware that allow for the recording of events or the collection of data. These peripheral devices are divided into two categories, medical peripherals and non-medical peripherals. Medical peripherals can be used only for medical purposes, while non-medical peripherals can also be used for other purposes.

Medical Peripherals

They either collect medical images such as those captured by an otoscope (for the ears), ophthalmoscope (for the eyes), dermascope (for the skin) or any other kind of medical imaging device. Other devices may increase bodily sounds. The most common device is electronic stethoscope by which specialist can listen to heart, lung and bowel sounds, while conducting a telemedicine examination over a videoconference system.

Then there are medical peripherals used to collect biometric data of patient like pulse, blood pressure (BP), etc. Images from imaging devices such as echocardiogram, ultrasound, microscope and surgical devices, laparoscope, endoscope, etc. also can be transmitted using telemedicine. X-ray need to be digitized, hence there is need for digital X-ray processing machines.

Non-medical Peripherals

Many devices and instruments are used along with videoconferencing to assist in transmission of information and ideas. Many institutions use inexpensive, commercially available video cameras as an essential part of their telemedicine network. Another non-medical peripheral is the videotape recorder. A video can be made of a specific patient or procedure that would not be available at the time, a consultation is scheduled. Scanners used to scan and X-rays are also another such devices.

LIMITATIONS TO SPREAD OF TELEMEDICINE

Telemedicine however has its limitations. Some of these are listed below:

1. Poor patient-doctor relationships: This is most likely when paramedical staff or patients directly use telemedicine to get consultation and there is no direct contact. But this can be corrected by making the interaction of real-time and with adequate follow-up with the consulting doctor using email/telephone, etc.
2. Patient acceptance: It can be improved by adequately educating the patients and other users about the aims and benefits of the new technology.
3. Fear of technology: The technology is new and there will be apprehensions. Hence, all persons using this will need to be adequately trained. The trainers will need to be with the persons operating till they are adequately confident in using the machines.
4. Low rates of utilization: Initially, there may be a low rate of utilization and if run commercially, may not be viable. But, with increasing use as with anything new, the user base will pick up.
5. Infrastructure: Costly equipment needs to be put in place for starting telemedicine that too in places, where basic medical facilities do not exist. This will be the picture in developing countries. National policy and government support for use of telemedicine will need to be formulated. In India, this has not been put in place.

ETHICAL ISSUES

The most important ethical issues are the doctor-patient relationship, the confidentiality of patient data, the standard of care, the liability of the physician and physician's accreditation:

1. Circumstances when patients interact with doctors only through telemedicine links either directly or using paramedical staffs as intermediaries pose problems.

2. Patients feel that their data is not secure when being transmitted over electronic media. But this feeling can be overcome by using encryption of data and educating the patients about the use of secure means of data transfer, and also in reassuring the patient that data will not be made public at the other end where it is received. The clinician in direct contact must assume full responsibility for the confidentiality of patient data.
3. To ensure confidentiality of data, legislation is required. The United Kingdom (UK) Data Protection Act (1998) and Computer Misuse Act of 1990 give some guidelines on confidentiality of data.
4. Another issue is a physician not licensed in a particular region may offer telemedicine care and then the question of his/her liability in case of mismanagement arises. This issue has not been answered.
5. Also if a mishap occurs, what is the jurisdiction of the offence?
6. The liability of paramedical staff, offering telemedicine advice has also been questioned. Though in UK and United States of America (USA), the organizations offering telemedicine service have been held responsible for these issues, telemedicine services from other countries are still not licensed.

Telemedicine has thus raised many questions. But these can only be answered when more people start using these services and regulations are framed by medical associations of user countries. Awareness increases the responsibility of the providers, hence patients and users need to be educated properly.

INDIAN SCENARIO

Now with the availability of internet connection in most cities of India, interest in telemedicine is increasing day by day, but still major drawback in India is that communication network is not suitable for most telemedicine applications. ISDN lines are not available in most of the places in India, which is basic requirement for videoconferencing. So at present and for some time, videoconferencing technology will be limited to some big cities and telemedicine technology that will be used in most of the parts of India will be store and forward technology. It will be like sending radiological images, patient records, sounds through email or modem and getting opinion of experts.

Many medical centers in India are now successfully running telemedicine projects using videoconferencing. Future of telemedicine in India is definitely bright, with availability of internet everywhere, with new information technology policy and with improving telecommunication network; use of telemedicine is going to increase. India is an ideal place to use this technology as 80% population in India lives in villages, where treatment is provided by quacks and unqualified medical practitioners. So, if one can use this technology to serve village population in India that will definitely improve quality of medical care.

The internet has made possible an excellent method to provide accessible healthcare telemedicine. Telemedicine can improve the quality of care, provide medical access to previously inaccessible areas, helping in managing emergencies, in managing chronic illness and in providing health education all over the world; more so in developing countries where access to medical care is limited.

CONCLUSION

Technological advances through digital compression of data, voice and video images have created new avenues in the telemedicine, and have made the transmission of the data more acceptable in a cost-effective manner. Telemedicine with its improved and fullest applications would remodel the role of medical and health care, and work practices in the coming years. Health professionals, information technology scientists, the telecommunication sector and the government agencies need to work together to make the fullest use of this promising technology.

FURTHER READING

1. Department of Defense, USA. [online]. Telemedicine. Available from http;//www.tatrc.org/
2. The European Health Telematics Observatory. [online]. Available from http://www.ehto.be
3. Federal Telemedicine Gateway. [online]. Available from http://www.cbloch.com
4. Freeman k, Wynn j, Groves-Phillips s, et al. Teleconsulting: a practical account of pitfalls, problems and promise. Experience from TEAM Project group: Telemed Telecare. 1996; 2(Suppl 1):1-3.
5. Bauer JC, Ringel MA. Telemedicine and the Reinvention of Health care. Newyork: Mc-Graw-Hil; 1999.
6. Darkins AW, Cary MA. Telemedicine and Telehealth: Principles, Policies, Performance and pitfalls. London: Springer; 2000.

7. Editorial. Time Magazine. 1998;52(2):20.
8. Goldstien DE. e-healthcare. Harness the power of Internet, e-commerce and e-care, Aspen, Gaithersburg, MO, 2000. In: Wotton R, Craig J (Eds). Introduction to Telemedicine. London: Royal Society of Medicien; 1999.
9. Thacker N, Vidyashankar C. Telemedicine. In: Thacker N (Ed). Computers for Doctors. New Delhi: Jaypee Brothers Medical Publishers (P) Ltd; 2003. pp. 127-42.

18

Application of Computers in Nursing

Lincy John, Naveen Thacker

Science has bestowed health care delivery system with excellent technological innovations. One such innovation is the computerization of the entire health care delivery system. Computerization has contributed enormously towards the reduction of medical errors and the problems associated with such errors (Gan et al., 2005). Computerization of health care delivery includes computerization of the medical records popularly known as the Electronic Medical Record System (EMR), Electronic Prescriptions, Personal Digital Assistants, Computer Automated Cancer Detection and Computerized Theatre Management Applications. Computers are used in different aspects of nursing.

Computers in nursing education: Even in the field of nursing education, computers help the tutors/educators to present the large and complicated data, which of course is a part of the medical study, in a very simplified and effective format. Features such as PowerPoint presentations, slide shows, videos, enable a better understanding of the complex medical procedures and more.

Nursing education must involve a lot of practice programs to make the students efficient to face the real-life scenarios. Computer programs enable simulate such procedures, thereby being of great use.

Computers also contribute and help the students know their strengths and weaknesses. There are many quiz programs and medical tests with immediate feedback that can help you brush and develop your medical facts and requirements, without any delay. Your queries are solved, you know the answers, and you know where you stand. A regular use of such computer applications definitely make you more equipped and well-researched for your field.

The most appealing and outstanding feature of computer-based education is that it gives a boost to interactive learning. Unlike traditional methods of learning, where everything was done based on papers and individual understanding, computer-insisted learning encourages more interaction and communication among the instructors and the students, thereby increasing the scope to learn and understand better.

Computer in nursing practice: Nurses must spend a considerable amount of time documenting the care they are giving to their patients. In non-computerized environments, this involves writing the nursing notes in longhand. These notes report on the treatments, medications, procedures, diagnostic tests, and other components of the patient's health and activity over a certain period of time. In computerized environments, the documentation process can be automated through the use of standard reporting forms and checklists that allow the nurse to use various computer interface modalities to quickly enter the information concerning the patient. Menus, windows, pointing devices, or cursor keys can be used to select standard items from lists, while specific data (such as numeric values) can be entered via a keyboard. This automated documentation process not only saves time, but it also increases the accuracy of patient information and makes it more readily accessible for diagnostic or statistical analysis.

Computerized patient care planning can be implemented in a manner similar to the documentation process noted previously. Since standard lists of nursing diagnoses and interventions for particular patient problems have been prepared for almost all areas of nursing, it is not too great a leap to present these items via computer, so that they can be selected and associated with particular patients.

Another big area of computer application in health care with major implications for nursing functions is patient monitoring. Dedicated computer controlled devices have been utilized for bedside monitoring of electrocardiogram, heart and breathing rate, temperature, and various other vital physiological parameters for over 10 years. Presently these systems are becoming much more sophisticated and they are being integrated with the automated recordkeeping mentioned previously. In this way, the monitored status of the patient becomes associated with the nursing and medical records entered by members of the health care team. In addition to this, automatic posting of laboratory test results keeps the record current and further reduces nursing paper work (previously, lab reports would pile up on the desk until filed away in the patient's chart). In all, this automated and integrated patient record becomes a powerful tool for patient monitoring, recordkeeping, ongoing assessment, and evaluation.

Nursing administration: Nursing administration is defined as the act of managing nursing duties, responsibilities, or rules. An example of administration is the act of the manager in the hospital managing the nursing staff and employing the rules of the health system.

Impact of computers in nursing administration can add a dimension of information that has not been provided by the traditional managerial methods. Computers are used in the administrative areas of nursing for basic tasks that once were done on paper. Staffing and scheduling systems are used to construct daily, weekly or monthly schedules. Many scheduling systems also collect data on individual employees such as the amount of sick time used or vacation hours accumulated. Staffing and scheduling systems often provide a variety of reports to the administrative nurse. Budgeting and financial tracking are another way in which computers are used in nursing administration.

FURTHER READING

1. How are computers used in the Nursing profession? http://work.chron.com/computers-used-nursing-profession-3402.html
2. What is the importance of computers in Nursing? https://www.reference.com/business-finance/importance-computers-nursing-381a18f9da59287c
3. Computers in Nursing Education, www.cybercorp.net/rhiggins/thesis/higlitd.html

Index

Page numbers followed by *f* refer to figures.